Carotid and Vertebral Artery Dissection

A Guide for Patients and their Loved Ones

Jodi A. Dodds, MD
Vascular Neurologist at Duke University
Founder of and Primary Contributor to *The Stroke Blog*

Amanda P. Anderson, MS, CCC-SLP
Speech-Language Pathologist
Carotid Artery Dissection Survivor

Cover: MR-angiogram image of a dissection of the left internal carotid artery and bilateral dissections of the vertebral arteries in their V1 and V2 segments

About the Authors:

Jodi A. Dodds, MD is a vascular ("stroke") neurologist and an assistant professor of neurology at Duke University. Her clinical work and research focuses on issues that impact the young adult stroke population. She is also the creator of and primary contributor to *The Stroke Blog*, which features information relevant to young stroke patients (http://strokeblog.net).

Amanda P. Anderson, MS, CCC-SLP is a speech-language pathologist who works with stroke survivors during their rehabilitation. She is the author of the *Speech Therapy Aphasia Rehabilitation (STAR)* workbook series and co-author of *Aphasia Recovery Connection's Guide to Living with Aphasia*. She is the recipient of the National Stroke Association's 2015 Raise Award for Outstanding Individual, and is a survivor of an internal carotid artery dissection.

We dedicate this book to the patients navigating through the aftermath of carotid and vertebral artery dissection, as well as their loved ones who strive to understand and cope with "the new normal."

Table of Contents

Introduction 1
Preface: The Balloon 9
Chapter 1: Blood Flow to the Brain 19
Chapter 2: *Patient Story: Circle of Willis* 33
Chapter 3: Carotid and Vertebral Dissection 39
Chapter 4: *Patient Story: Triple Threat* 71
Chapter 5: Diagnostic Tools 79
Chapter 6: *Patient Story: The Adjustment* 97
Chapter 7: Causes 107
Chapter 8: *Patient Story: A Couple's Perspective* 133
Chapter 9: Initial Treatment 143
Chapter 10: *Patient Story: Successful Intervention* 159
Chapter 11: Pain 163
Chapter 12: *Patient Story: Exhausted* 191
Chapter 13: Aftermath Symptoms: 195
Chapter 14: *Patient Story: Finding Support* 207
Chapter 15: Life After Dissection 213
Afterword 245
Acknowledgements 249

Disclaimer: This book is intended to be used for informational purposes only and should not be a substitute for advice from your medical provider. Never make any changes to your medical plan of care without discussing your care with your medical provider.

Introduction:
Why a Book Like This is Overdue

Patients with carotid and vertebral artery dissections (also known as cervical artery dissections because they occur in arteries traveling along the cervical spine) are some of my very favorite individuals to treat for many reasons. Among them, the vast majority of the time, if they are correctly diagnosed before a stroke has occurred and are started on an appropriate medication, we are able to prevent a stroke. A research study ("The Cervical Artery Dissection in Stroke Study," or "CADISS") examined the medical treatment options for patients with carotid or vertebral artery dissections. Out of 150 patients presenting with very recent carotid or vertebral artery dissections, only four ended up having subsequent strokes after starting appropriate medication.

This fact is worth emphasizing again: **146 out of 150 patients with vertebral and carotid dissections did *not* have a stroke once diagnosed and treated.** Unfortunately, though, because patients with cervical artery dissections are frequently misdiagnosed or are not treated in time, they have strokes or even die in severe cases.

A cervical artery dissection (a "tear" or "rip" in the lining of a carotid or vertebral artery in the cervical spine, or neck) places a patient at higher risk for stroke. Throughout this book, we will use the terms "carotid and vertebral dissection" and "cervical artery dissection" interchangeably.

Neurologists are used to seeing what I have come to call the *aftermath* of stroke, which means that something bad has already occurred, and the focus of treatment must shift to managing symptoms and deficits resulting from the event. Making an accurate diagnosis of a carotid or vertebral artery dissection and treating it yields overwhelming odds that stroke can be prevented soon after treatment has started, which minimizes the aftermath.

Of course, patients also present for medical attention after a stroke has already occurred due to a cervical artery dissection. It is just as vital to identify and treat these to reduce the risk of a subsequent stroke.

Some of these cases are also among the saddest that I have seen as a vascular neurologist. As you will see in the patient story entitled "The Circle of Willis," the ending can be catastrophic. Depending on the circumstances, sometimes even the best medical care cannot save a life, largely due to what nature has bestowed upon a person long before a dissection has ever occurred.

The fact that patients with carotid or vertebral artery dissections are usually young and seemingly healthy makes it all that much more difficult when the outcome is not positive. I have seen patients with dissections in the same location within the same artery return to complete normalcy and others who do not survive.

Unfortunately, while some patients recover very well from cervical artery dissections, many survivors struggle with the aftermath of this vascular injury for years. In addition to pain, fatigue, and cognitive symptoms, they also face the stress of looking normal to the outside world, and because they appear normal, they frequently feel that they are expected by others to return to their previous level of functioning. Despite having the same external appearance, internally things have changed.

Over time, I have learned to schedule longer appointment times for patients with carotid and vertebral dissections, because I anticipate there will be numerous questions from both patients and their loved ones. Some of these questions have easier answers, and some I can only answer with: "We don't know yet." I say "yet," because I am optimistic that we will be able to provide answers someday with greater research efforts.

Some of the questions I have heard many dozens of times at this point include, but are not limited to, the following:

- Why have I coughed thousands of times in my life without a problem, but suddenly a cough three months ago dissected my artery?
- How did I push so hard through labor and delivery when my baby was born without dissecting my carotid artery, but when I sneezed, my artery tore?
- If warfarin (Coumadin) is "stronger" than aspirin, shouldn't I be taking that for my dissection?
- Why am I always tired if I didn't have a stroke?
- Why do I still have pain in my head and neck even though my scans all look normal now?
- Why have doctors said my symptoms are unrelated to my dissection?
- Why am I having panic attacks and insomnia if all of my scans now look okay?
- What is wrong with my short term memory since my dissection?
- Will I have another dissection in the future?
- How often should I have a CT-angiogram or MR-angiogram to check on my dissection?

- Is it safe to have another baby someday?
- Can I still safely have sex?
- Is this a genetic problem, and are my kids at higher risk for dissection?

I have often wished that someone knowledgeable in this area would write a comprehensive guide for patients and their loved ones about carotid and vertebral dissections so that I could distribute copies to my own patients who are struggling with dissection aftermath. Such a book never emerged.

Amanda Anderson, a speech-language pathologist and carotid artery dissection survivor who entrusted me with her care in 2011, contacted me over the New Year's Day holiday in 2016, stating that she needed a new project to take her mind off of the daily pain she had been experiencing since her dissection had occurred. She had already successfully turned pain into productivity and patient advocacy, creating a useful and badly-needed workbook series to assist patients with aphasia in their rehabilitation process, as well as authoring a book about aphasia recovery. She expressed a desire to help patients who had experienced carotid and vertebral artery dissections, and I thought – yes! The time has come to write that comprehensive book for these patients and their loved ones in hopes of answering many of their questions. I knew that Amanda's passion for the topic after her personal experience, as well as her background as a speech therapist, would make her a wonderful writing partner.

I also knew that I would enjoy the writing process. I had begun authoring *The Stroke Blog* in 2014 in an effort to answer some of the more common questions I was hearing from young stroke patients, so it seemed like a natural transition to provide this additional resource.

We have attempted to make the book as complete as possible without overwhelming our readers. If you are interested in reading more in-depth about certain topics covered, I would encourage you to look at the endnote references provided, as these can serve as resources for you. Since patients and their loved ones have so many questions about this vascular injury, the book is organized in a question and answer format. A common paraphrased question from patients will introduce the topic and the information following it will provide the best answer based on available research and clinical experiences. We have also included true stories of patients. These have been written by cervical artery dissection survivors who have given permission to share their stories in this book, with one exception. I have written the tale of one man who did not survive, and his wife has been generous in permitting us to share this story in his memory.

I truly hope that this book is helpful to you as you navigate through cervical artery dissection aftermath. Know that you are not alone if you now carry this diagnosis, and that you are a part of a very engaged patient group connecting with one another through social media and support groups. Greater understanding of what has occurred can promote emotional and psychological healing, and I hope this book is able to answer many of your questions.

- *Jodi A. Dodds, MD*

Patient Story:
The Balloon

As I hold a small opened bag of uninflated balloons in my hand, I experience mixed emotions. Anger, sadness, disbelief. I kept the rest of the balloons, evidence perhaps of my last day without pain, or a memento of what happened. Keeping these symbolic balloons seems silly, because I have enough daily reminders of that day without them.

I was a healthy mother of two beautiful little girls. I loved to run and had completed 13 marathons in 12 different states. I had hoped to run one in every state. That changed over five years ago, when I was 32 years old, in a simple and somewhat ridiculous way.

I was attempting to blow up a balloon for a Halloween party. Despite multiple attempts to blow up the balloon, it didn't budge. I kept trying and stupidly didn't give up. As I was struggling to blow up the balloon, I felt as if a bomb suddenly exploded inside my head. It was as if my eardrum had ruptured, but in a location deep within my skull. I remember thinking, "Wow, I'm going to have a headache later." Who knew that I would still be battling a severe daily headache over five years later.

About a week later, I started to experience scary symptoms. After a run on my treadmill, my vision in my right eye became distorted and the peripheral vision on my right-hand side became hazy, as though a half moon section of my visual world had vanished. I experienced a sudden, severe, piercing headache above my right eye, and my left arm became numb. The pain in my head was undeniably the most excruciating pain I had ever encountered, even worse than the two complicated deliveries of my daughters. The pain was relentless, leaving me helpless and unable to function.

After several hours of pain, persistent numbness in my arm, and nausea, my husband brought me to the ER. I had completely forgotten about the balloon incident a week earlier and had no idea what was wrong.

After waiting for several hours in the ER as I continued to combat agonizing pain, nausea, visual abnormalities, and now difficulty moving my left arm, I underwent a CT scan of my head. I was diagnosed with a migraine and discharged home.

Oddly, my symptoms did resolve for a few days, but they returned with a vengeance. Approximately one week following the ER evaluation, I awoke with a thunderclap headache above my right eye, left-sided tongue numbness and tingling, the half-moon of decreased vision, and severe nausea with vomiting. Since many of those symptoms are also associated with a migraine, we did not rush back to the ER.

The pain continued to be absolutely unbearable throughout the day, and when my left arm began to lose sensation again, I sought help from my primary care physician. It was Friday, and she ordered an MR-angiogram of the brain for Monday to evaluate blood flow in the arteries of the brain.

That evening the pain, nausea, numbness, and visual symptoms grew even worse. My husband took me back to the ER where I received a CT-angiogram, an imaging study that evaluates blood flow in the arteries. I had already had a CT scan during my first ER trip, but that did not evaluate blood flow - only the brain tissue itself.

Once the radiologist interpreted my scan, the ER doctor entered the room to talk to my husband and me. First, he asked if I had been in a car accident or ridden any roller coasters recently. I had not. Then he explained that I had torn the lining of my right internal carotid artery. He drew a picture with a large flap in my artery, explaining that the artery's lining was blocking blood from flowing to the right side of my brain.

My initial reaction wasn't panic, but relief. I was glad to have an explanation for my symptoms and ready for any procedure that could fix me.

Suddenly, doctors and nurses began to flock around me and gave me heparin to thin my blood. They started to treat me with great urgency, and I was emergently transported to the hospital downtown to their specialized neuroscience unit.

The next week in the hospital was a blur of MRIs, IVs, and different medications to attempt to prevent stroke and to alleviate the pain. My husband spent the week by my side and slept on the hospital room couch while our family looked after our daughters. I felt as though an ax had buried itself in my head. I hallucinated, felt light-headed, and was disappointed and confused when I learned there were no surgical options that would fix me. I did not think I would be able to manage any aspect of my life if the pain did not stop.

My dissection was in a location that would have made a stent (a device designed to hold an artery open) placement risky without guarantee of benefit. My dissection flap, or the tissue that had separated from the wall of my carotid artery, was also completely blocking blood flow, which would have presented large obstacles in trying to place a stent. The right side of my brain was borrowing blood from the left side and back of my brain until the issue could stabilize. The doctors that saw me kept telling me how lucky I was to be alive.

The dissection had completely incapacitated me with pain and I didn't have the energy to sit up, much less the fight to recover. If I had not received medical attention, I truly believe I could have slipped away.

Fortunately, my daughters went to preschool with the children of a pediatric neurologist, Dr. Stephanie Robinett. My husband called her and asked if she knew anyone who could help. Her friend and colleague, Dr. Jodi A. Dodds, was a vascular neurologist (stroke specialist) and the medical director for neurosciences at the hospital where I was an inpatient. Dr. Robinett called Dr. Dodds that evening, and immediately from home Dr. Dodds began looking at my scans and started to direct my care and saved me from a stroke, and in my opinion, saved my life.

I felt like I was drowning, and when Dr. Dodds called me that night, I was rescued. She calmly explained what had happened to my internal carotid artery and how my other arteries were able to compensate and supply my brain with blood. She recognized my pain, understood my fears, and discussed with me medical options for treatment. She showed me empathy, patience, kindness, and respect.

My blood pressure had been running very low, and when it dropped, I became confused, my left arm went numb again and my vision became blurry. As my blood pressure dropped, my TIA symptoms returned. Part of my early treatment involved bringing my blood pressure up to a normal range, and when it was normal, my symptoms were substantially better.

Over the following five years I struggled with only having the energy for little things. A trip to the grocery store would exhaust me for two days. Background noise became painful, and going out to a restaurant or the movies became too overwhelming. To this day, every day my head and body feel as if I have I a massive hangover with nausea, sensitivity to light and sound, with a constant crushing headache.

At the six month mark, I had a follow up MR-angiogram. Because I had been feeling so awful, I didn't think my carotid dissection had improved, but to my surprise, the artery was actually open. I had restored blood flow to my brain again, and at least from the standpoint of what was present on the MR-angiogram, my artery had healed well.

Dr. Dodds has always been honest and upfront with me. When I sought a second opinion to see if a neurosurgeon would recommend a stent or even surgery, she encouraged me. The neurosurgeon agreed with Dr. Dodds' plan of care and said that stenting in my particular case was dangerous and unnecessary. I have learned that excellent doctors welcome questions and understand the need to seek multiple opinions. When my preventative pain medication stopped working, I made appointments with other doctors hoping for a cure. There is very little information available for patients about what to expect after experiencing a cervical artery dissection.

I have heard a variety of explanations about why I continue to struggle with symptoms even though my artery has opened up again. I've heard some pretty trite explanations such as stress, anxiety, and sadly some doctors have told me that I am not in pain and insist that my symptoms don't exist. One doctor even suggested that I take a stress management class. I am not in pain because I experience stress. I am stressed because I am in pain!

I am fortunate. My immediate family, especially my husband, is extremely supportive and understanding. Also, I love the work that I do. I am a speech-language pathologist and work with stroke survivors. If I had any other job, I don't think I would be able to continue working. I work in a quiet environment with the elderly.

Sometimes I mourn my old self. I'm sad that I miss out on participating in activities with my children and family. Some of my life plans to travel and run a marathon in every state have slipped away.

After my dissection, I initially had difficulty with word-finding. I also had trouble understanding what others were saying. It took me a few extra seconds to process information, especially if there was any background noise. Although I didn't have a stroke and no damage presents itself on my scans, I still have many of the post-stroke symptoms, such as fatigue, anxiety, difficulty concentrating and pain.

I empathize with my speech therapy patients who have had severe strokes with aphasia. Aphasia impacts a person's ability to speak and understand language. After my dissection, I created a series of workbooks to help people with aphasia with their recovery.

I took a copy of my first workbook to my next appointment with Dr. Dodds, and she enthusiastically told me that there was a huge need for a tool like this for stroke survivors with aphasia who wished to work towards language recovery. She encouraged me to write more workbooks and at the time of publication of this book, I have published a total of four workbooks in the *Speech Therapy Aphasia Rehabilitation (STAR)* series and co-authored *Aphasia Recovery Connection's Guide to Living with Aphasia*. My carotid artery dissection has increased my compassion for stroke survivors and motivated me to help make a difference for individuals with aphasia. Because of my pain, I am less physically active, but I have had the time to become an author, which I might not have done if I had never blown up that balloon.

If you are still struggling to come to terms with the changes that cervical artery dissection brings, keep in mind that perhaps your path will now be different than the one you had always imagined.

From participating in support groups with other survivors of cervical artery dissection, I know others haven't been as fortunate. We are told we are lucky to be alive, but we are still dealing with the aftermath of the dissection. Of course we are grateful and feel extremely blessed to have survived, but it is challenging, to say the least, to adapt to pain, exhaustion, cognitive impairment, anxiety, and to have to put on hold many of our life plans.

Survivors of carotid and vertebral artery dissections are frequently left with many unanswered questions. To date, there has not been a single resource for patients that is comprehensive and aims to cover the full spectrum of questions that patients and their loved ones may have.

Dr. Dodds and I collaborated on this book in an effort to answer many of those questions. Most importantly, we believe that survivors need to know that they are not alone struggling to live with the symptoms of their dissections. We wrote this book to share information and current research so that survivors and their families can better understand this diagnosis.

- *Amanda P. Anderson, MS, CCC-SLP*

Chapter 1:

Blood Flow to the Brain 101

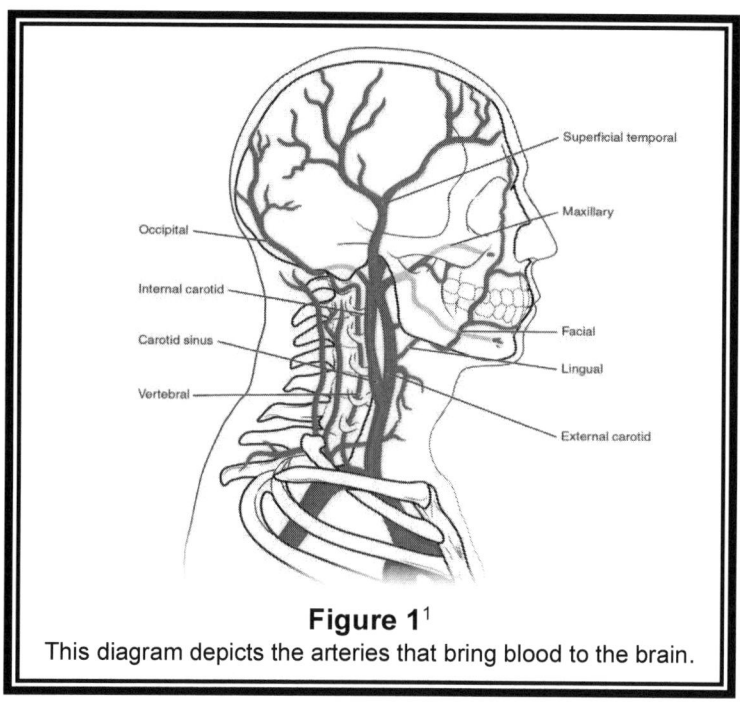

Figure 1[1]
This diagram depicts the arteries that bring blood to the brain.

"How does the brain receive the blood that it needs?"

There are four major arteries in the necks of the majority of people that bring oxygen-rich blood to the brain. We use the words "majority of people" here because some people are born with only three! These arteries are essential to supplying the brain with oxygen. Without a steady stream of oxygen, brain cells die, resulting in an ischemic stroke.

"What is an ischemic stroke, and how common is it?"

Ischemic strokes result when blood clots or other abnormal structures (plaque, for example) block blood flow to the brain, and cells in the brain die from the lack of oxygen. Ischemic strokes comprise approximately 87% of all strokes, with hemorrhagic strokes (bleeding) accounting for the remaining cases.[2] Depending on the location within the brain and extent of damage to these brain cells, disability and even death can occur.

Stroke is the leading cause of disability worldwide. According to the World Health Organization, 15 million people per year have a stroke. Of these 15 million strokes worldwide, roughly five million people die and another five million are permanently disabled. The CDC reports that in the United States, one American dies from a stroke on average every four minutes.[3] Although 75% of stroke cases are in individuals over 65, 25% or 3.75 million strokes a year in individuals under 65 worldwide.

"Is there a difference between the carotid and vertebral arteries, and the 'cervical arteries'?"

The carotid and vertebral arteries are known as cervical arteries because they travel adjacent to the cervical spine in the neck. As mentioned in the Introduction, throughout the book when we refer to both the carotid and vertebral arteries, we may use the term cervical arteries. Cervical arteries in our necks have nothing to do with the cervix of the uterus. Many research studies use the term cervical arteries, and for those interested in reading available information about dissection, it is necessary to understand the term cervical arteries.

"What are the carotid and vertebral arteries and what is their role in bringing blood to the brain?"

The two main arteries in the front of the neck are the common carotid arteries. There is one on the right side and one on the left. If you find your pulse in the front of your neck with your fingers, what you are feeling is a carotid artery expanding and contracting. Below the mandible, or jaw, the common carotid artery splits into two branches: the internal and external carotid arteries. It is the internal carotid artery that carries blood to the brain.

The two arteries traveling towards the brain in the back of the neck are the vertebral arteries, appropriately named as they maneuver through openings in the transverse processes of the cervical spine vertebrae. When it was mentioned earlier that some people are born with only three major arteries traveling through the neck to bring blood to the brain, we meant that some only have one vertebral artery. In these cases, the single vertebral artery is larger than normal to accommodate for the additional blood it needs to carry. Most people do not ever realize they possess this anatomical variant, and their brains receive the blood flow that is needed without incident.

A very common scenario is for a person to have a dominant vertebral artery. In this case, two vertebral arteries are present, but one vertebral artery is larger than the other. The smaller artery may be hypoplastic, or less well-developed. If you find that you have a dominant vertebral artery and a hypoplastic vertebral artery, the dominant vertebral artery is usually able to pick up the slack from the smaller vertebral artery and there shouldn't be any cause for alarm.

The vertebral arteries come together once they are inside of the skull to form the basilar artery. The latter parts of the vertebral arteries and the basilar artery supply blood to the brainstem and cerebellum.

The brainstem controls the most essential functions to sustain life, including breathing, heart rate, blood pressure, and swallowing, to name a few, in addition to enabling us to move our arms and legs. We must have brainstem function in order to survive, and for most people, it is critical that blood flow continues through the basilar artery for this purpose. The fact that two arteries join together to create the basilar artery, as opposed to the basilar artery arising as a branch of another artery, tells us how vital this blood vessel is. If a vertebral artery becomes blocked, blood flow usually still continues in the basilar artery through the unaffected vertebral artery that remains open. Nature protects us with this beautiful redundancy!

"How is blood distributed once it enters the brain?"

Because a constant supply of oxygen-rich blood is so essential to the brain, there are safeguards in our anatomy to better ensure that the brain receives the blood that it needs. A constant oxygen-rich blood supply is achieved in part by arteries coming together in a traffic circle called the Circle of Willis.

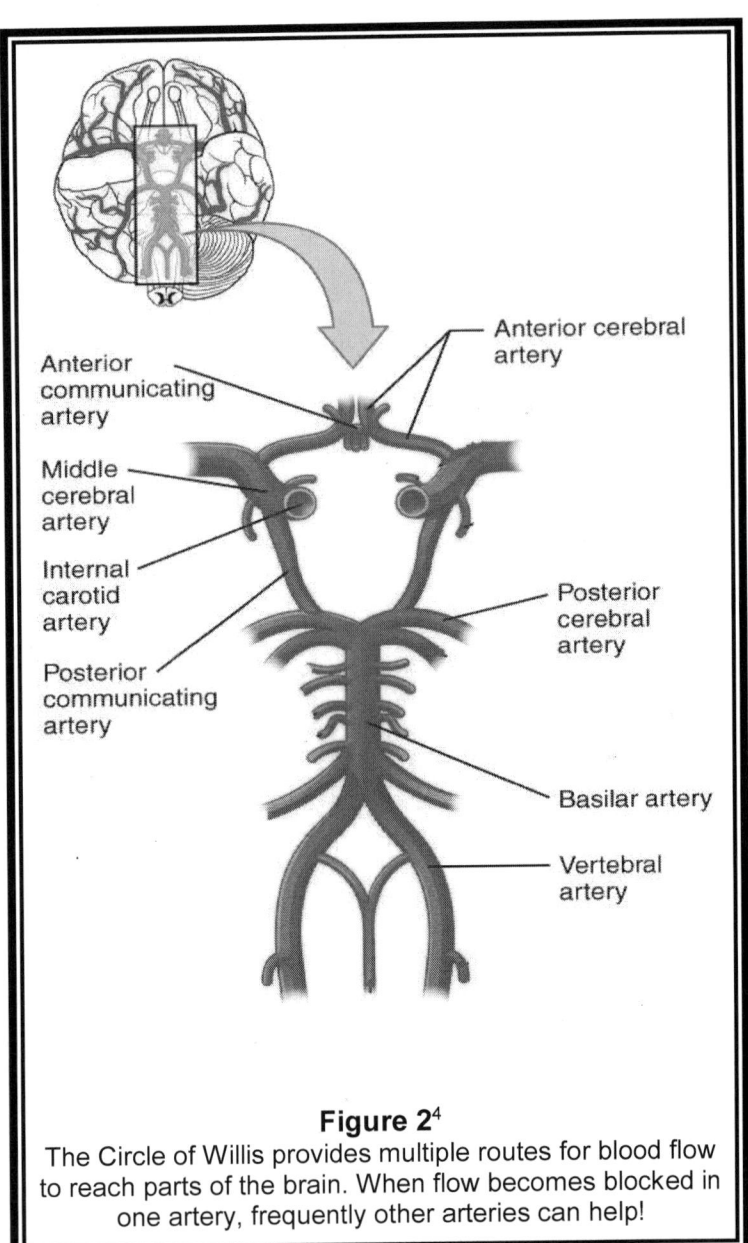

Figure 2[4]
The Circle of Willis provides multiple routes for blood flow to reach parts of the brain. When flow becomes blocked in one artery, frequently other arteries can help!

If you refer to Figure 2, you should see that all four of the cervical arteries (two internal carotid arteries and two vertebral arteries) travel to the base of the brain. Once in the brain, the major arteries that extend from the internal carotid arteries are the middle cerebral arteries (one on each side). The middle cerebral arteries supply blood to approximately 2/3 of each half of the brain, or each cerebral hemisphere.

Smaller arteries supplying the inner midline surfaces of the brain also arise from the internal carotid arteries, called the anterior cerebral arteries. In the majority of people, there is a bridge between the right and left anterior cerebral arteries across the midline of the brain, called the anterior communicating artery, nicknamed the "AComm." With the AComm comes a connection in blood flow between the right and left sides of the brain.

Just as there is an AComm connecting the right and left halves of circulation in the brains of many people, the posterior communicating arteries, or "PComms," connect blood flow from the vertebral arteries and basilar artery from the back of the brain to the front, and vice versa.

"**My carotid artery is blocked on one side. I have never had a stroke, but I'm concerned. Why isn't my doctor worried about this?**"

In some people, a carotid artery occlusion, or blockage, can occur and no symptoms will be present. The side of the brain with the blocked internal carotid artery is borrowing blood from the other side where the internal carotid artery is still open, using what is called collateral flow. Perhaps the blood-sharing is occurring through an amazing AComm.

There is also the potential for sharing blood between the back of the brain and the front, via posterior communicating arteries, nicknamed "PComms," potentially one on each side. A complete Circle of Willis is present in people with both an AComm connecting the right and left halves of the brain's circulation as well as two PComms connecting blood flow in the front to the back on both sides. Anywhere from 25-42% of people possess a complete Circle of Willis, meaning that an AComm and two PComms are present, completing the traffic-circle. Meanwhile, the remaining individuals may lack one or multiple collateral vessels.[5,6]

For example, a person may have an AComm, but no PComms, and another person may lack both an AComm and PComms.

Ideally, if any of the cervical arteries have restricted blood flow within them, the other arteries can start to supply blood to brain cells in need and prevent a stroke from occurring.

The AComm is approximately four millimeters in length, which is about the height of four thin coins stacked together. Though it is quite small, the presence or absence of an AComm can mean the difference between a major stroke and death versus no neurological symptoms at all after a dissection.

Figure 3 is another image of the Circle of Willis from a different viewpoint (looking at the base of the brain). You can see the circular shape to this structure.

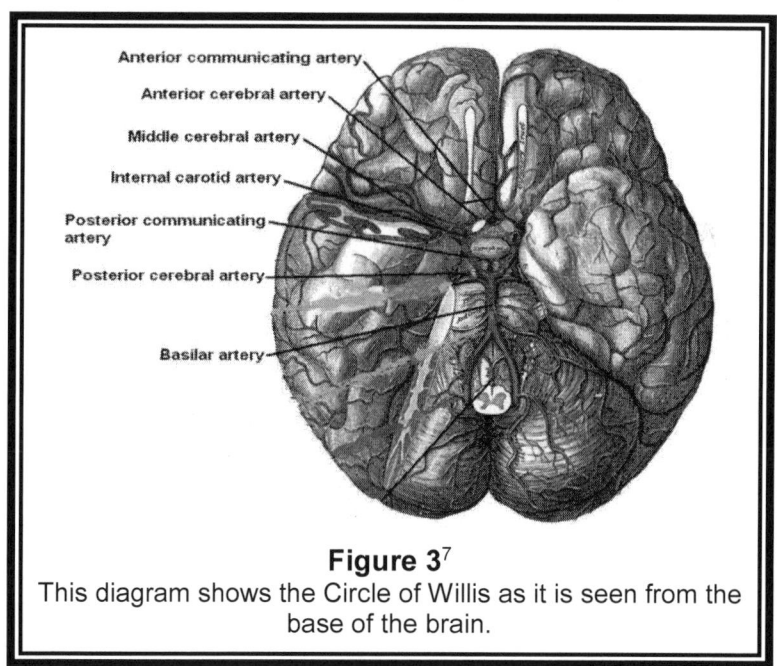

Figure 3[7]
This diagram shows the Circle of Willis as it is seen from the base of the brain.

"I have been diagnosed with a dissection in one of the arteries in my neck. What is that exactly?"

In order to understand what a dissection is, it is first necessary to understand what gives an artery its structure. The cervical arteries are made up of three layers of tissue, which are diagrammed in Figure 4.

The *tunica intima* is the innermost layer of the artery and is smooth, thin and fragile compared to the other layers of the artery. The tunica intima is sometimes referred to as an "onion-skin layer" that lines the inside of the artery. It is composed of endothelial cells, which have direct contact with the blood stream, and a thin layer of connective tissue.[8]

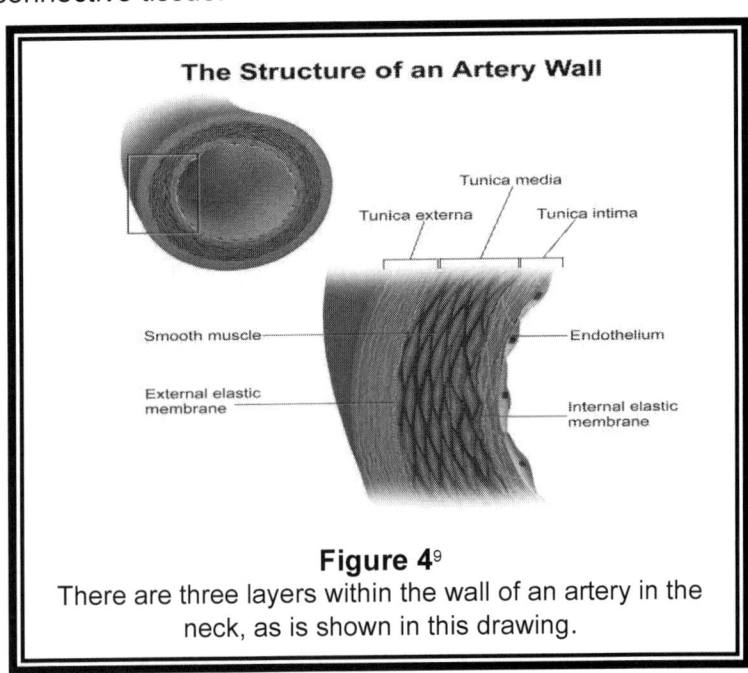

Figure 4[9]
There are three layers within the wall of an artery in the neck, as is shown in this drawing.

The middle layer of the cervical arteries, or *tunica media*, is the thickest layer and able to make autonomic (involuntary) contractions to regulate the size of the artery. The smooth muscle of the tunica media allows for vascular constriction and dilation to help regulate blood pressure and body temperature.

The outermost layer of the cervical arteries is the tunica adventitia, comprised of strong and flexible collagen fibers. Collagen fibers are cables used by our bodies in building connective tissue. The tunica adventitia also connects to bone surfaces in order to anchor arteries in place.[10]

A cervical artery dissection occurs when the inner lining of the artery (tunica intima) in either a carotid artery or a vertebral artery segment in the neck separates from the rest of the artery. Another way to describe this is that a section of the endothelial layer tears from the rest of the arterial layers, creating a flap that can cause narrowing or occlusion in the artery.

"Are there differences between carotid and vertebral artery dissections in the neck and dissections that occur in arteries in the brain?"

Yes, there are differences. When an artery traveling in the neck enters the *dura* (one of the layers of thin tissue that covers the brain), the artery becomes thinner. The strong outer tunica adventitia layer of a vertebral artery, for example, thins as the vessel passes through the dura within the skull.[11] If a vertebral or carotid artery in the neck dissects spontaneously or as a result of relatively minor trauma, the vessel is very unlikely to rupture due in large part to the fact that the adventitia is thick and strong. Damage to an artery in the neck is usually confined to the inner layer(s) of the artery. An intracranial dissection (inside the skull) may be at a higher risk of rupture because the adventitia is not as thick and supportive of the vascular structure.

"How does blood pressure factor into this?"

The contraction of cervical arteries is directly related to contractions of the heart. As the heart beats, the arteries contract to push blood to the brain and other organs. In general, the more constriction present in arteries, the harder the heart has to work to pump blood, and the higher the blood pressure will be. Some medications that treat hypertension (high blood pressure) work by relaxing the arteries so that they are not as constricted.

A normal blood pressure for a healthy adult is around 120/80 mmHg. The systolic pressure (the top number) is a measurement of the amount of pressure present in pushing blood forward as the heart is contracting. The diastolic pressure (the bottom number) measures the pressure in your arteries when your heart is resting between contractions.

When narrowing is present in an artery - and in particular an artery supplying blood to the brain, such as a carotid or vertebral artery - the blood pressure may be elevated partially because more pressure is required to push blood through the narrowed area, and partially because the brain is commanding this flow if it is not receiving enough blood. When a person is having an ischemic stroke, it is likely that blood pressure will be elevated. Often, doctors treating ischemic strokes within the first few days utilize permissive hypertension by allowing the blood pressure to remain high in order to optimize blood flow to the brain.

"How do veins differ from arteries?"

Both the purpose and the structure of veins differ substantially from arteries. Arteries carry oxygen-rich blood to our organs, while veins bring blood that has already delivered this oxygen back to the heart.

The wall of a vein is thin compared to that of an artery and does not contract as forcefully. The primary reason for the difference in wall thickness is that the amount of pressure within an artery is much higher than it is in a vein. As blood flows through arteries, then to arterioles, then to capillaries, then to venules, and finally to veins, the amount of pressure propelling blood flow falls substantially. Thick walls are not necessary to contain blood by the time it flows through veins.

Chapter 2: Patient Story
A Tale of Two Carotid Artery Dissections, and the Miracle of the Circle of Willis[12]

(Published on *The Stroke Blog* in October 2014)

In Memory of Edward Ritch

Nature is kind to some, and not so merciful to others. With this thought in mind, I try to reflect daily and be thankful to have enjoyed another day with my family, friends, and patients.

I have seen patients arrive with completely blocked carotid arteries and absolutely no symptoms, and when evaluating cerebral blood flow with ultrasound or with angiographic imaging, it is clear that the side of the brain with the carotid artery occlusion is borrowing blood from the other side, using what is called collateral flow. There is the potential for sharing blood between the front of the brain and the back, via posterior communicating arteries (PComms, potentially one on each side). There is also potential for sharing blood flow between the right and left hemispheres of the brain via the anterior communicating artery, AComm. A complete circle of an AComm and two PComms in addition to the other normal arteries in the brain is known as a complete Circle of Willis. About 30% of people possess a complete Circle of Willis.

During a weekend when I was on call, a previously healthy man in his 40s transferred from an outside hospital for management of an extensive right hemispheric ischemic stroke. He was critically ill upon arrival with an extremely concerning neurological exam. His imaging of his arteries revealed that he had a right internal carotid artery dissection with thrombus (clot) obstructing flow. The right hemisphere of his brain was ischemic, and he was unable to generate alternative ways of obtaining blood flow to this region in his brain. He lacked a complete Circle of Willis – no AComm and no PComms.

I find that certain days exist in which neurological themes declare themselves. On some days, I will see four patients consecutively who all have atrial fibrillation, an irregular heart rhythm that can result in ischemic strokes. On other days, I may receive three referrals for stroke that occurred during pregnancy or in the postpartum period. On that particular weekend, though, the theme was clearly carotid artery dissections.

As I was leaving this man's room in the neurological intensive care unit, the ER paged me, requesting guidance on a woman who had arrived with drooping of an eyelid (ptosis), and her pupil on the same side was more constricted than in the eye on the other side. The description sounded like a classic case of

Horner syndrome. Horner syndrome can occur with an injury to the internal carotid artery, which can result in both of the findings mentioned, as well as abnormal sweating on the affected side of the face.

I recommended that the patient have a brain MRI along with an MR-angiogram of the head and neck to better exclude the possibility of a carotid artery dissection, a potential cause of Horner syndrome. I received a page soon after this that her imaging was, indeed, consistent with a significant right internal carotid artery dissection. Fortunately, there was no stroke present. Aside from the eyelid droop and abnormally sized pupil, she was completely neurologically normal despite having complete occlusion of her right internal carotid artery from her dissection. Her MR-angiogram of the brain revealed that she possessed not only a nearly identical dissection in the same vessel as my other patient, but she also had something valuable that the first patient lacked – **she had an AComm.**

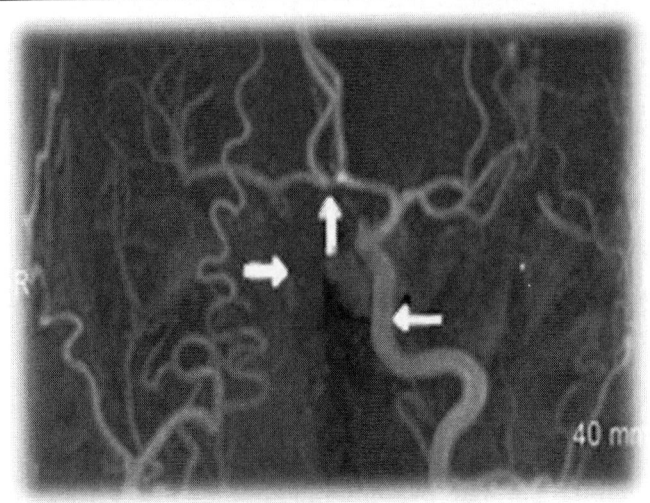

Figure 5
The patient's MR-angiogram image illustrates the AComm successfully providing blood flow from the left side of the brain (on your right side) to the right (your left). There is no flow in the right internal carotid artery due to a dissection.

The arrow on your right delineates flow in this patient's normal left internal carotid artery. (We are facing the patient with this orientation, so what is on our right is actually the patient's left side, and vice versa.) The arrow on your left demonstrates the absence of blood flow in the right internal carotid artery. The top arrow identifies the AComm, connecting the left (normal) circulation in the brain to the right side, which enabled the patient to avoid a stroke.

When I evaluated the patient, she told me that she became concerned about the abnormal appearance of her pupil and had decided to seek medical attention for this in the ER rather than waiting until Monday to talk to her primary care provider. She was started on antiplatelet therapy for stroke prevention. Nearly one year later, her Horner syndrome had improved (although not completely resolved), and she was doing well, having never sustained a stroke.

I am convinced that carotid artery dissections are underdiagnosed. Frequently, these patients present to the ER or to their primary care providers with headaches that seem like migraines at first glance. Perhaps a head CT scan is performed, which is not an effective study for excluding ischemic stroke (especially very early stroke). A brain MRI is a more sensitive tool for identifying early ischemic stroke, but if a carotid artery dissection is present, it will only be seen on a brain MRI if the dissection is located close to the brain or is large enough to limit blood flow. If the dissection is small, or located farther down in the neck, a brain MRI will miss it. If a patient seeks medical attention for a severe headache unlike any other previously experienced, a migraine that differs from the patient's description of his/her typical migraines if the person is already a migraine sufferer, or if the patient has any associated neurological symptoms involving the face, eyes, speech, or extremities, a brain

MRI along with some sort of imaging of the arteries in the head and neck should be performed.

I reflect back on the ironic juxtaposition of these two patients presenting on the same morning and marvel at what a difference the presence of a tiny artery in the brain can make. In this case, it was the difference between returning to a good, normal life without stroke, and tragically in the first patient's case, an untimely death. He developed severe swelling within the brain following his stroke, and despite aggressive medical and neurosurgical intervention, he passed away within the week.

I have often wondered if I have a complete Circle of Willis. Do I have an AComm? I don't know. I do not have an answer, and perhaps I will never seek one, because what is up there is working for now, and I cannot change what I have. Certain cards are dealt to us long before we ever take our first breaths in the world, and as much as we like to feel empowered to create our own destinies, we do not have a say in whether our Circles are complete or not. Stroke brings the realization of a loss of control, and with this comes fear and anxiety. Stroke is more than just a diagnosis with symptoms. But when I see a patient with a carotid artery dissection and an Acomm providing flow, I see perseverance, and it gives me pause.

Chapter 3:
Carotid and Vertebral Artery Dissection

"I have been diagnosed with a cervical artery dissection. What is this?"

As discussed in Chapter 1, a cervical artery dissection occurs when one of the inner vascular layers of a carotid or vertebral artery segment in the neck forcefully separates from the remaining outer layers. Most commonly, the intima (the "onion-skin" thin layer of endothelial cells) separates from the media and adventitia. The inner layer tears away from the thicker, more robust layers of the artery.

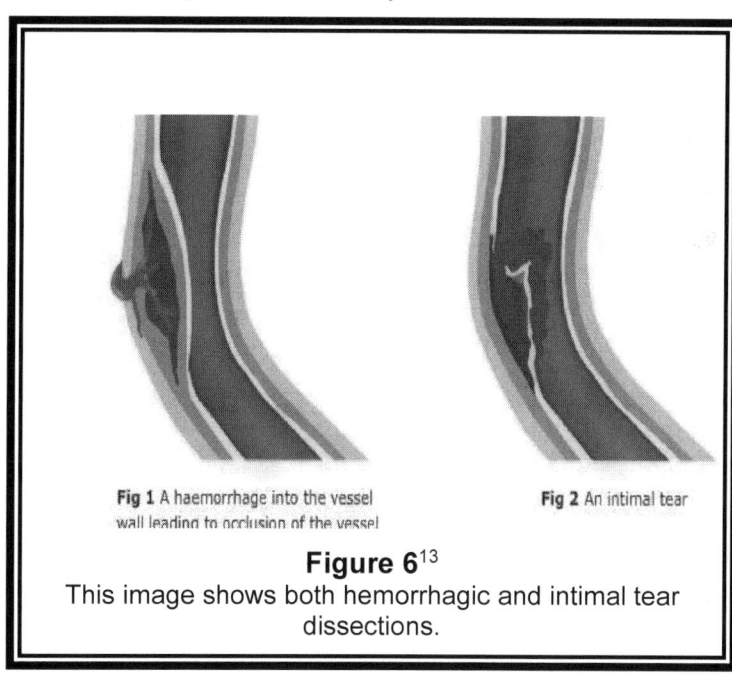

Fig 1 A haemorrhage into the vessel wall leading to occlusion of the vessel

Fig 2 An intimal tear

Figure 6[13]
This image shows both hemorrhagic and intimal tear dissections.

Vascular dissections can affect intracranial (inside of the skull) or extracranial (outside of the skull) arteries. In fact, any artery can be dissected. Dissections of the aorta can be catastrophic if they are severe enough. They can also cause strokes.

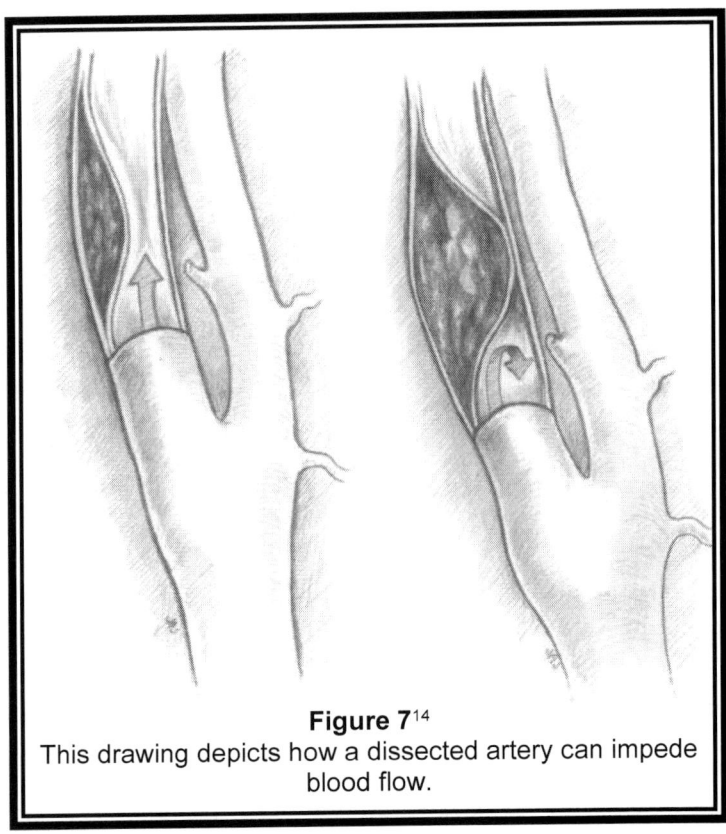

Figure 7[14]
This drawing depicts how a dissected artery can impede blood flow.

Bleeding can also occur within the wall of the artery. When bleeding into the arterial wall takes place, this collection of blood is known as a mural hematoma. In severe dissection, the tissue flap and clot formed within the arterial wall may create a complete occlusion, or blockage, of blood flow (Figure 7). In the absence of a flap, bleeding can occur between vascular layers in this space, forming a bulge (mural hematoma), which in turn may also cause narrowing or occlusion of the artery (Figures 6 and 7).

"How common are carotid and vertebral artery dissections?"

We suspect if a random survey were taken of adults on a busy street corner asking about familiarity with the terms "carotid artery dissection" or "vertebral artery dissection," most people would likely never have heard these terms. However, these arterial injuries account for up to one quarter of ischemic strokes in young adults.[15]

Cervical artery dissections have an annual incidence cited at about three people per 100,000.[16] This assumes, of course, that all cervical artery dissections are diagnosed. Because the condition is likely underdiagnosed, the exact incidence is probably unknown. We suspect it is higher.

A number of patients with cervical artery dissections will never know that they have them because symptoms will either be mild or nonexistent, or perhaps the diagnosis is missed. They may present with neck pain and a headache that fades over several weeks. If a stroke never occurs, this event may be diagnosed as a migraine, "neck strain," tension headache, concussion, or other more common ailments.

Carotid artery dissections are more common than vertebral artery dissections, with about two people in every 100,000 presenting with carotid artery dissection and one in every 100,000 with vertebral artery dissection on an annual basis.[17] However, as will be discussed later, vertebral artery dissections can be more challenging to diagnose than carotid artery dissections, so these numbers are also questionable.

The average age of individuals at the time of a cervical artery dissection is 45. Dissections occur slightly more frequently in males than females.[18] In children under 18, dissections tend to occur predominantly in boys, possibly due to risky physical activity and resulting trauma.[19] Also, cervical artery dissections tend to be more prevalent in the fall or winter months, which could be related to cold and flu season and subsequent coughing and vomiting, well-documented causes of these vascular injuries.[20]

It wasn't until the 1970s that carotid and vertebral dissections could be diagnosed using vascular imaging. Before that, carotid and vertebral dissections were only discovered post mortem during autopsies.[21] Although the diagnosis of carotid and vertebral dissection is relatively new because of advances in imaging technology, people have probably been experiencing dissections for thousands of years and living with symptoms, with no explanation for them.

"I know someone who had narrowing in an artery because of plaque buildup, but my artery is narrow because of a dissection. How are these two conditions different?"

It is important to understand the difference between carotid artery disease due to atherosclerosis and carotid artery dissection. Atherosclerosis results from the accumulation of plaque in the wall of an artery and occurs in carotid and vertebral arteries, as well as in the coronary arteries that supply blood to the heart. Risk factors for the development of atherosclerosis overlap with a number of well-documented stroke risk factors:

- Cigarette smoking
- Hypertension
- Diabetes mellitus
- Hyperlipidemia (high cholesterol)

- Obesity
- Obstructive sleep apnea

Many people refer to atherosclerosis as "hardening of the arteries." As plaque accumulates, calcium begins depositing in the wall of the artery. Calcium is the same element that provides the rigid structure to our bones and teeth, so, indeed, this condition results in literal "hardening" of the arteries.

Another distinction between atherosclerosis and carotid and vertebral dissections is that with plaque obstruction, the plaque can be removed surgically. An endarterectomy physically removes plaque from the artery with the goal of restoring blood flow. After a dissection, it isn't possible to simply remove the blockage because the blockage is created by a bulge or flap in the arterial lining.

Unlike vascular disease due to atherosclerosis, cervical artery dissections are not related to these more familiar stroke risk factors. In fact, there is an inverse relationship between obesity and high cholesterol and the risk for carotid and vertebral dissection.[22] In other words, the healthier you are with respect to body weight and cholesterol, the higher your chances are of having a cervical artery dissection, even if the absolute risk is not very high in the general population.

A dissection results from the separation of vascular layers within the arterial wall. The narrowing that can result in an artery is due to the "onion-skin" endothelial tissue "flap" dangling from the artery wall and blocking some or all of the blood flow in that vessel. Blood flow is reduced or blocked in people with atherosclerosis by plaque buildup, not by a tissue flap or bulge.

"Wait a minute - patients with cervical artery dissections are usually healthier people? Can that be right?"

People with cervical artery dissections are younger, less likely to smoke, and less likely to have diabetes than stroke patients without dissections.[23] Many cervical artery dissection survivors report that they sustained their dissections when they were in good physical shape. The sudden onset of a serious vascular injury may make patients feel especially vulnerable. The event is frequently unexpected.

"Why are cervical artery dissections concerning?"

The substantial concern for healthcare providers in a patient presenting with an acute cervical artery dissection is the increased risk of stroke. As was explained previously, an ischemic stroke occurs when a portion of the brain does not receive the blood flow needed to sustain its functions. When brain cells do not receive oxygen for even a few minutes, they will die. Brain cell death results in a permanent brain injury. If blood flow returns to the brain before cell death has occurred and a person's stroke-like symptoms completely resolve, this is known as a *transient ischemic attack,* or TIA. Sometimes patients ask – what is a TIA called when the brain *is* damaged? The answer is – a stroke.

"How do cervical artery dissections cause strokes?"

Most strokes that occur as a result of cervical artery dissection are not due to blockage of the carotid or vertebral arteries themselves, although this certainly can be the mechanism for a stroke if the brain is not able to "borrow" blood flow from other sources. The brain does a marvelous job of borrowing blood from alternative sources when these vessels are occluded.

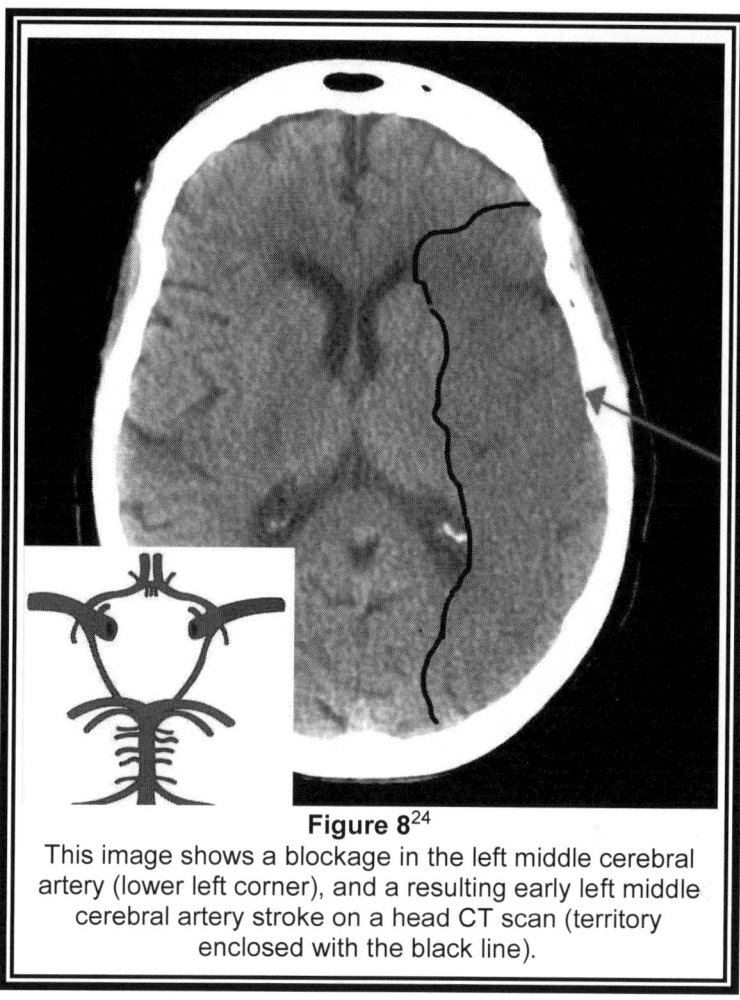

Figure 8[24]
This image shows a blockage in the left middle cerebral artery (lower left corner), and a resulting early left middle cerebral artery stroke on a head CT scan (territory enclosed with the black line).

Figure 8 shows an occlusion just outside of the Circle of Willis in the middle cerebral artery, which resulted in a large ischemic stroke. The more frequent mechanism of stroke in cervical artery dissections involves emboli. Emboli are blood clots, vascular debris, and platelets that break loose from the injured blood vessel wall, travel from the dissection site to an artery downstream from that site, and lodge within that vessel, blocking blood flow. When the artery wall is traumatized, platelets collect in the inflamed dissected tissue. Because many of these artery branch points where emboli travel and block are outside of the Circle of Willis, it can be more challenging to obtain alternative sources of blood flow, resulting in ischemic stroke.

"I was diagnosed with a TIA and also a 'mini-stroke.' What are these and are they actually strokes?"

A Transient Ischemic Attack (or TIA) occurs when blood flow is disrupted to the brain and symptoms concerning for stroke occur. In a TIA, blood flow is either restored or the brain compensates for the absence of blood flow by seeking and acquiring blood from other sources and *no damage to the brain occurs*.

There is some misconception about what a transient ischemic attack really is. The mainstream media and even some medical professionals have referred to a TIA as a mini-stroke, a term that has become very popular in our culture, and is heard all of the time by neurologists from patients and their family members:

"It was just a slight mini-stroke."

"Aunt Rose had a mini-stroke while eating."

"He had a touch of the mini-stroke."

A stroke is a stroke. Period. A stroke results in an injury to the brain. There are two basic types of strokes – ischemic and hemorrhagic. An ischemic stroke occurs when blood cannot reach part of the brain for a prolonged period of time and permanent damage to brain tissue takes place. A hemorrhagic stroke takes place when a blood vessel ruptures and bleeding occurs within the brain. Approximately 85% of strokes are of the ischemic type.

During a stroke, brain damage occurs. During a TIA, damage does not occur. What about a TIA during which damage *does* occur? What is that called? The answer is – a stroke. To describe a TIA as a "mini-stroke" misses the difference between the two terms. A TIA is not a stroke because damage is avoided. A stroke is not a TIA because brain damage has occurred. A TIA is an *almost*-stroke, as opposed to a *mini*-stroke.

Sometimes patients inaccurately refer to a stroke with relatively mild deficits as a "mini-stroke" to distinguish it from a stroke that leaves someone physically disabled. However, some patients without a single physical visible deficit from a stroke are significantly disabled from the cognitive impairments that frequently result after a brain injury.

Once upon a time, there was a patient whose only symptom from her "mini-stroke" (her term) was left-sided neglect syndrome, where the brain fails to recognize that the left side of the body exists, even though the left arm and leg may move appropriately and strength on the left side can be left fully intact. She was a successfully employed person prior to her stroke, and she has not been able to work since her stroke. She does not factor in columns on the left half of the screen when working with spreadsheets because her brain fails to recognize the left half of her conceptual world. She neglects to brush the left side of her hair and has tooth decay in the left side of her mouth because she does not brush her teeth on that side. She cannot drive because she visually neglects cars that appear in the left half of her world, even though her vision on the left side is intact. Is this really a *mini*-stroke?

Perhaps the other reason why we prefer to avoid the modifier "mini" in front of a word as significant as "stroke" is because patients tend to downplay the importance of the event. Caring for patients after TIAs is a privilege, because damage to the brain has not yet occurred, and healthcare providers can still intervene to prevent a stroke. If a patient has a TIA and refers to it as "mini," then there may be less motivation for the person to quit smoking, comply with medication use, make healthy dietary changes, or exercise regularly. After all, it was only a *mini*-stroke.

"I read online about 'dissecting aneurysms.' How are these different from cervical artery dissections?"

An aneurysm is an abnormally dilated segment of a blood vessel.[25] If there is significant weakness in the wall of the artery at this dilated segment, an aneurysm can become larger and can even rupture, resulting in bleeding. Cerebral aneurysms are aneurysms that occur in the arteries of the brain.

A dissecting aneurysm occurs when the arterial layers separate at the site of aneurysm, as opposed to a cervical artery dissection, where the layer separation occurs in a neck segment of an artery where there is no aneurysm present. Dissecting aneurysms in the brain can result in a hemorrhage if the outer lining of the artery tears completely.[26]

After a cervical artery dissection (again, this is a dissection occurring in the neck, not the brain) occurs, there may be a pseudoaneurysm or a *dilation* of the dissection site on follow-up imaging. As one might suspect, "pseudo" means "false," so these are not true aneurysms in the sense that they are at relatively low risk for rupture. Cervical artery dissections typically result from a tear between the inner layer (tunica intima) and possibly the middle layer (tunica media) of a cervical artery.[27] If the tough outer layer of the artery (tunica adventitia) is unscathed, then despite some dilation or stretching of the vessel at the dissection site, the vessel is still strong, and the risk for rupture is relatively low.

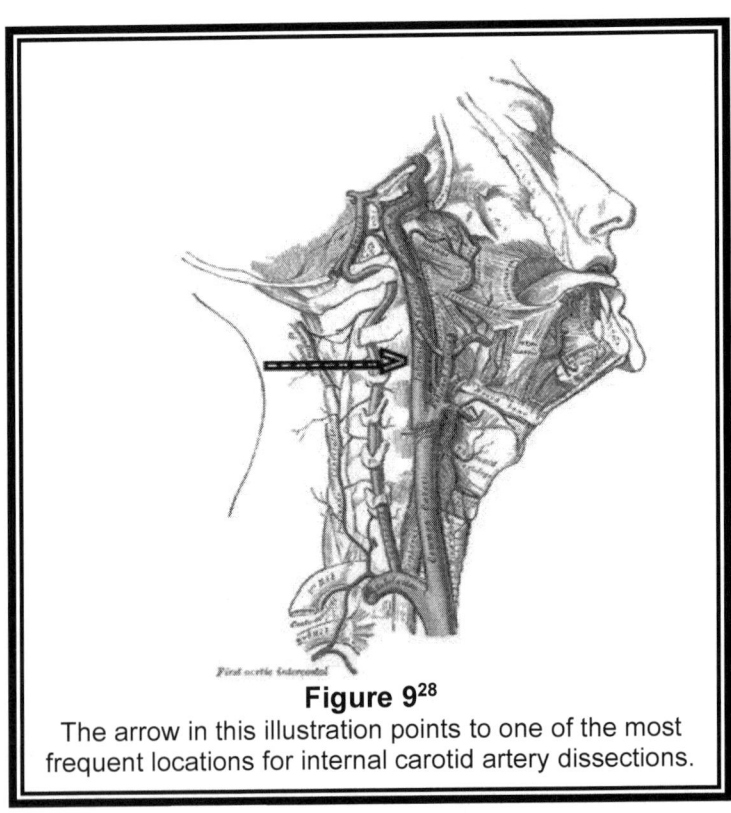

Figure 9[28]
The arrow in this illustration points to one of the most frequent locations for internal carotid artery dissections.

"In which parts of the carotid and vertebral arteries are dissections most common?"

Carotid artery dissections occur most often in the internal carotid artery approximately two centimeters above the bifurcation (split) of the common carotid artery into the external and internal carotid arteries. The arrow in Figure 9 shows approximately where the most frequent site of internal carotid artery dissection occurs above the bifurcation of the common carotid artery. This segment in the internal carotid artery above the bifurcation is near the base of the skull.

Dissections at this location comprise about 2.5% of all first-time strokes.[29] Although 2.5% sounds low, it actually translates to approximately 15,000 strokes a year in the United States alone. The internal carotid artery travels over the cervical spine vertebrae C2 and C3, which makes this location vulnerable to injury with sudden movement or sudden neck extension that pushes the artery against bones of the cervical spine.

Vertebral artery dissections most frequently occur between cervical vertebrae C1 and C2. C1 bears much of the flexing and extending the neck. Vertebral artery dissections also occur between C5 and C6, where the artery initially enters the transverse foramina (holes) on both sides of the cervical spine.[30] Figure 10 demonstrates cervical spine flexion and extension on an x-ray and also is labeled to demonstrate the position of each cervical vertebrae.

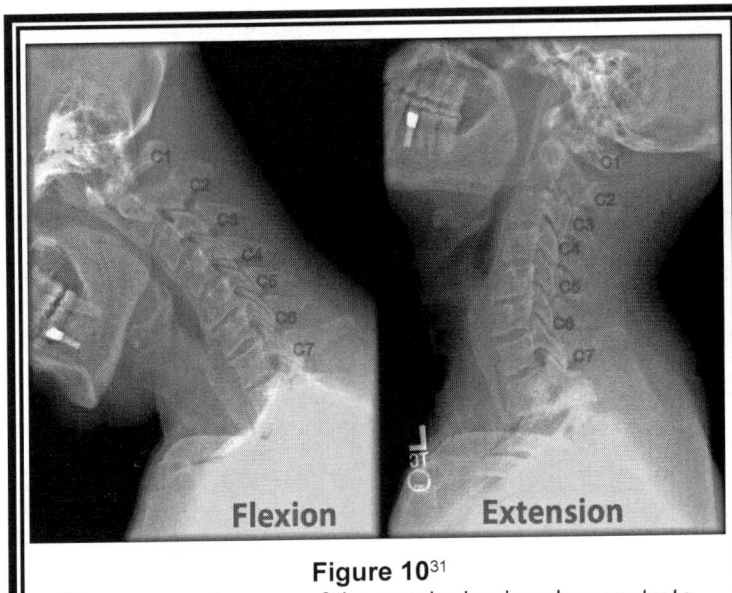

Figure 10[31]
These x-ray images of the cervical spine demonstrate flexion and extension.

"How does a person know that he or she has a cervical artery dissection? What are the symptoms?"

When people experience carotid or vertebral dissections, they may present with a variety of symptoms, many of which may be incorrectly attributed to another more common condition such as migraine or hypoglycemia (low blood sugar levels). Cervical artery dissection is frequently misdiagnosed early in its course.

Initially, patients with cervical artery dissections may present with one or some of the following symptoms:
- Neck pain
- Headache (which can range from mild to severe)
- Pupils that are not equal in size, and possibly accompanied by drooping of an eyelid
- Vertigo
- Fainting
- Nausea and/or vomiting
- Visual loss, either affecting vision in one eye or half of the vision when looking with either eye
- Paralysis and/or numbness on one side of the body if there is already reduced blood flow to a portion of the brain, brainstem, or cerebellum

Neurological symptoms may not develop for a number of days following a cervical artery dissection. Because of the potential lapse in time between when nonspecific pain first develops and when focal neurological symptoms more concerning for stroke begin, there is usually time to accurately diagnose the dissection and to start treatment in order to prevent disabling or potentially fatal results.[32]

Headache is one of the most common symptoms for individuals who experience a carotid or vertebral artery dissection. One study found that emergency departments report headaches being present in approximately 75% of cervical artery dissection patients.[33] As many as 92% of patients with carotid artery dissections present with a headache in the emergency department, and up to 72% of patients with vertebral artery dissections present with headaches.[34] The headaches can be intense, and they may be referred to as "thunderclap" headaches if the pain is very sudden and severe in onset. Pain can also center around the jaw and the ear. Facial, scalp, and neck pain are also common complaints. However, the absence of neck pain does *not* indicate the absence of a cervical artery dissection.

Slurred speech, difficulty with word finding (aphasia), and impaired swallowing may also be present. Taste disturbances and even tongue numbness on one side can result from cervical artery dissection. If the brain can compensate by using other arteries to supply enough oxygen-rich blood, neurological symptoms may not ever occur.

"I don't think my vision has been the same since my dissection and stroke. I have trouble explaining exactly how my vision has been affected. What is going on?"

Vision impairment is a common acute symptom of carotid and vertebral dissections and is a red flag that brings many people with dissections to the ER. Visual deficits following a brain injury tend to fall into one of the categories outlined below. While scores of neurological conditions can result in these visual syndromes, for our purposes we will keep the focus on stroke and dissection.

- **Diplopia**, or double vision, occurs when more than one image of an object is visualized by the patient. Most commonly, it occurs because the eyes are not aligning properly to fixate on a visual target, and as a result of failing to converge at a specific point, mixed visual information is presented to the brain. When a patient has experienced a stroke, most often the injury was in the brainstem because there are centers controlling eye movements in this location. Double vision can also occur if there is an injury to one of the cranial nerves controlling eye movement closer to the eye itself, even if the brainstem is not injured.

- **Visual aura** often is described as "blurry vision" by patients, but it is much more complex than this description would suggest. Stroke patients may experience temporary visual illusions, such as the visualization of distorted surroundings, blurring of a crescent-shaped area or a larger section in a person's visual world, flashing lights, wavy lines, development of "tunnel vision," or any other number of transient visual symptoms. Fortunately, visual aura is benign and treatable in most cases. Patients may be concerned that episodes of visual aura are TIAs that may represent the start of another stroke. Some patients have been taking warfarin or other big-gun anticlotting therapy for years because of "TIAs," but ultimately it turns out to be visual aura.
- **Homonymous Hemianopia** occurs when a visual field is distorted or absent, meaning that one half of someone's visual world is impacted. Often patients will think they have lost vision in the right eye or in the left eye, but testing reveals that the eyes are fine, but half of the person's visual world is absent which typically occurs with an injury to the occipital lobe, the brain's visual processing center. Put simply, the right occipital lobe processes visual information in the left field

of vision, and the left occipital lobe processes the right field. A stroke impacting the right occipital lobe may result in loss of vision in the left visual field, and vice versa.

- **Visual Hallucinations** occur when a patient detects objects or movements that are not actually present. Visual hallucinations can occur for a variety of reasons, involving either the brain or the eye. Charles Bonnet syndrome is the name given to visual loss followed by the brain "filling in" missing visual information in the form of hallucinations. The hallucinations may be pleasant (a cuddly kitten), or they may be disturbing (large insects). If visual hallucinations are present after a stroke, it is worth performing an electroencephalogram (EEG) during the hallucination, if possible, to better exclude seizure activity in the area of injury.
- **Oscillopsia** is present when a patient perceives that objects at rest are "swaying" back and forth when movement is not actually present, and can occur with brainstem or cerebellar stroke, but it can result from injuries to other locations as well. Patients without stroke may experience this visual phenomenon with benign paroxysmal

positional vertigo ("inner ear" vertigo, as a lot of patients describe it) or with migraine as well.
- **Cortical Blindness** typically involves injury to both occipital lobes. Patients lack vision, even though the eyes are usually healthy. The sudden loss of vision can be devastating for patients, as these are typically patients who have always relied on vision and who abruptly become blind quickly since stroke is usually of sudden onset. To make things even more challenging, some patients with cortical blindness develop Anton Syndrome, which involves blindness without the recognition that blindness exists. Can you imagine everything around you seeming real, but none of what you are visualizing is actually there?

Finally, there is blurry vision. Regardless of the stroke's location, patients often complain that their glasses prescription does not seem correct any more. They may obtain a new prescription after the stroke, only to find that it is no longer accurate six weeks later. A neuro-ophthalmologist (a neurologist or an ophthalmologist who specializes in visual symptoms after a brain injury) can be helpful here, but it takes patience from both patient and physician as symptoms tend to fluctuate.[35]

"When I was in the hospital with my dissection, the doctors and nurses wouldn't let me eat or drink anything at first. Why?"

Patients with stroke are at higher risk of aspiration when trying to eat or drink because their swallowing function may be impaired, and food or liquids could end up in the lungs instead of in the stomach. More severe cases of dysphagia (impaired swallowing) can result in aspiration pneumonia from food or liquid entering the airway rather than traveling to the esophagus/stomach and falling into the lungs, placing the patient at risk for infection.

Cervical artery dissections can damage cranial nerves that control swallowing function, or swallowing can be impaired if stroke has occurred. Coughing is your body's way of protecting your airway. If there is cranial nerve damage and subsequent muscle weakness, you are at higher risk for having food and liquid falling into your airway. If you cough after you eat and drink and have a wet vocal quality during or after eating, these are signs that your swallow function may be impaired.

Initially in the hospital, typically a nurse will perform a brief evaluation to determine whether there are signs present that you might be at risk for aspiration. Some of these signs include slurred speech and/or a facial droop. If this first screen indicates that swallowing could be impaired, usually you will be made "NPO" status ("Nothing By Mouth") until a speech-language pathologist (SLP) has evaluated you more comprehensively. If uncertainty about swallowing function remains after this bedside assessment, then the speech therapist may request additional tests, such as a modified barium swallow study or FEES (Fiberoptic Endoscopic Evaluation of Swallowing).

A modified barium study (MBS) uses real-time x-ray called fluoroscopy. The test is performed by a radiologist and an SLP. The SLP provides patients with substances of different consistencies mixed with barium. Barium is white, safe to consume, and shows up on an x-ray. This test will determine if anything enters your airway when you swallow. Often thin liquids are the most difficult to swallow after a stroke because they travel quickly, and the body needs time to close the epiglottis to block liquids from entering the airway. The SLP determines what consistencies can safely be swallowed and may adjust your diet to reduce the risk of choking and aspiration pneumonia.

Your SLP may choose to use a FEES (Fiberoptic Endoscopic Evaluation of Swallowing) to evaluate your swallow function as well. This test uses an endoscope, which is a flexible tube with a small camera and light on the end of it. The endoscope is connected to a computer that will display a live video of the vocal cords and other structures in the throat as swallowing takes place. The endoscopic tube is inserted through the nose and down the back of the throat. Patients are given different consistencies mixed with food coloring (usually blue) to make it easier to see while swallowing is viewed on the monitor.

"I kept hearing a 'whooshing' sound before I was diagnosed with my carotid artery dissection. What caused this symptom, and should I be worried?"

Hearing a ringing sound that is not resulting from an external source in the environment, or tinnitus, and hearing "whooshing" sounds corresponding with your pulse (pulsatile tinnitus) may be present in individuals with cervical artery dissections. As many as 25% of patients with dissections present with pulsatile tinnitus.[36] The whooshing sound is likely caused by increased pressure and speed of blood flow at the narrowed arterial site with each heartbeat. The flow at that site is likely turbulent.

Think of how water flowing smoothly in a small river sounds. Now think of how water in this same river sounds if the bank becomes jagged and narrow, with rocks strewn across the narrowing, making the bottom of the river bumpy and irregular. These conditions create rapids, and rapids within blood are essentially what occurs when blood is flowing through a tight, irregular space. A bruit is the sound that can result when the turbulence can be heard through a stethoscope by another party.

Since we like analogies, please consider another one. Narrowing in an artery can be compared to a garden hose through which water is flowing. Picture what happens to the water's flow as the hose becomes pinched off if there is a kink in it. As the inside of the hose narrows, more pressure builds at the site just before the narrowing. The speed at which the water is flowing also increases just before the narrowing, because the increased pressure pushes the water along more rapidly.

Often, narrowing in a carotid artery is "high-grade," or greater than 70%, for pulsatile tinnitus to be present (but not always!). Degrees of pulsatile tinnitus can vary. Some individuals experience a loud "whooshing" sound constantly, which can be extremely distracting and exhausting for the person enduring it. Others may only hear it when they lie down on the side of the dissected artery or after increased activity. The sound can vary depending on the size and location of the dissection. Some patients report hearing a light clicking sound.

"I was diagnosed with Horner syndrome along with my carotid artery dissection. What is that?"

Approximately one-third of patients with carotid artery dissection present with Horner syndrome.[37] Horner syndrome can also result from vertebral artery dissections; one study found that 36 out of 269 (13%) patients with vertebral artery dissections had Horner syndrome.[38] Horner syndrome is a group of neurological findings that are present following an injury to the sympathetic chain (the group of autonomic nerves that travel alongside the carotid artery that create our "fight-or-flight" responses). These findings include pupils that are unequal in size, drooping of the eyelid on the eye with the smaller pupil (and on the same side as the dissection), and decreased sweating on the same side of the face as the smaller pupil with the drooping eyelid (ptosis), as illustrated in Figure 11.[39]

A dissection can cause a rip through the sympathetic nerve chain and direct trauma to the nerve fibers. Nerve fibers of the sympathetic chain and cranial nerves travel alongside and adhere to the cervical arteries. Nerve fibers can also tear along with the lining of the cervical artery from a dissection. Different nerves are impacted depending on where the dissection occurs. In some patients, the nerves will heal and regenerate (nerves can do this outside of the brain and spinal cord), but in others, if the trauma to the sympathetic nerve chain is too severe, the symptoms will persist.

So why are these particular findings with the pupil, eyelid, and sweating present? Here we should consider the fight-or-flight response. Our sympathetic nervous system triggers a series of involuntary neurological changes to prepare us for survival under extreme circumstances, when running from a bear that is chasing you in the middle of the night, for example.

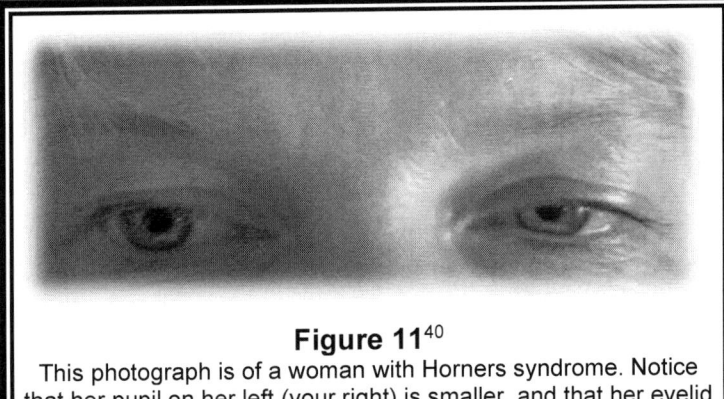

Figure 11[40]
This photograph is of a woman with Horners syndrome. Notice that her pupil on her left (your right) is smaller, and that her eyelid on that side is drooping.

In order to see clearly where you are running while it is dark, the pupil dilates and becomes larger, allowing more light to enter the eye. If the sympathetic supply to the pupil is interrupted, the pupil cannot dilate normally, which is why the pupil on the side of the sympathetic chain/carotid artery dissection is smaller in size.

In order to keep your eyelids from blocking your view while you eagerly watch your path as you run from this bear, your eyes open wider. When the sympathetic input is damaged, the result is an inability to open the eye fully, and the eyelid can droop.

While running, you begin sweating in order to keep your body temperature consistent and to prevent overheating. Without sympathetic input, however, sweating is reduced or absent to the region affected by the sympathetic chain injury.

If you have had a carotid dissection and are uncertain as to whether your pupils differ in size, try going into a dark room for a minute. If you are able to dim the lights the room, please do so, and look in a mirror at your eyes. If one pupil is dramatically smaller than the other, this is consistent with a possible Horner syndrome. The difference is more pronounced in the dark because the "good" pupil dilates to a larger size, but the pupil on the side of the carotid dissection remains small if the sympathetic chain was injured.

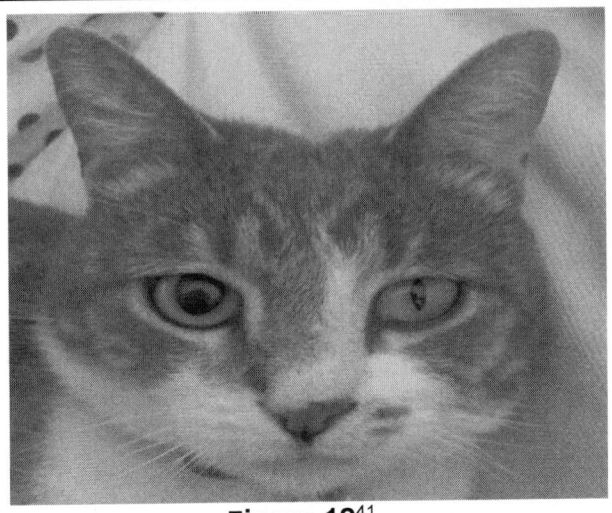

Figure 12[41]
This photograph depicts a cat with Horner syndrome. Again, notice that the cat's left pupil (on your right side) is smaller. Because of damage to the sympathetic chain on the cat's left side, that pupil is unable to dilate in dim lighting.

All symptoms of Horner syndrome may not be present when the sympathetic chain is injured from a cervical artery dissection. Many patients may have the pupillary asymmetry and the drooping eyelid, but facial sweating function may be intact.

Once blood flow returns in the artery when the dissection has healed, sometimes the symptoms of Horner syndrome gradually resolve. In other cases, despite having a healed artery, nerve damage remains after a dissection and Horner syndrome persists.

"I had a lot of nausea and vomiting with my vertebral artery dissection. Why would a damaged artery cause this?"

Both vertebral and carotid artery dissections can result in nausea and vomiting, especially when symptoms first start. Vomiting is a symptom that should be taken very seriously, in large part because it is a common stroke symptom. Restricted blood flow to the brainstem and cerebellum in particular (areas supplied by the vertebral arteries) can result in vomiting. Migraine may also occur as a result of carotid and vertebral artery dissections, and vomiting is a well-recognized part of the migraine syndrome. On the more frightening side of things, vomiting could indicate that the brain is swelling and that there is increased pressure.[42] Patients with recent dissections and severe, refractory vomiting should be monitored very closely in a hospital setting.

Chapter 4: Patient Story
Triple Threat

I had given birth to my second daughter only one week before. I went to bed that night and everything was fine, but I woke up with the worst pain I could have imagined across the top of my head. That's really saying a lot, since my daughter came quickly the week before, and I had an *au naturel* childbirth without an epidural or heavy pain killers! I would have taken the childbirth pain over this pain in my head any day! I also had loud whooshing (pulsatile tinnitus) in my ears. My neck felt swollen in the muscles on the sides.

    As a nurse, I knew something was very wrong. I went to the obstetrician (because in the postpartum stage, you initially see the OB no matter what is wrong). He said, "You have a lot of stress. You have a newborn and a toddler. You probably aren't sleeping well. Of course you have a headache." He sent me home. I could not lie down because the pain was so severe. I could not bear for the lights to be on. I could not tolerate any noise whatsoever. I was miserable and I knew this was not "just a headache."

    A few days passed. I went back to the OB's office and I was seen by a different doctor. I made up my mind I would not leave the office until something was done. I could not live like this. He said he would send me to a neurologist. By the time I was able to be seen by a neurologist, an entire week had passed, and I almost cancelled the appointment because the pain had subsided significantly. I did end up going, and the neurologist seemed concerned and said I needed an MRI as soon as possible. It was scheduled for the next afternoon.

My husband drove me to the MRI, and afterwards he took me out to dinner since we already had a sitter for our kids. I thought that surely, they would not have let me leave the MRI center if there was anything terribly wrong, so I didn't worry, and we went about eating our dinner. That night would be the last night things would ever be normal for us again.

The next day, I was home caring for my toddler and newborn when the neurologist called me and asked if I was home alone. She told me to call my husband to come home from work immediately, chew up an aspirin, and lie down because I was likely going to have a stroke. I needed to be admitted into the hospital immediately. I had dissected both of my internal carotid arteries. One was 75% blocked and the other was 99% blocked. I could not believe what I was hearing. As a cardiovascular nurse for 12 years, I was quite certain that I would not be alive if this were true. There must be some mistake! At this point, nine long painful days had passed since the onset of my symptoms. I needed to be home to take care of my kids. Instead, I spent two nights in the hospital where I was started on a lot of medication for my blood pressure, which was out of control due to the dissections. I was also started on coumadin, a blood thinner, for stroke prevention. I was discharged on Sunday afternoon and told to "go home and live (my) life. This was a fluke and it will never happen again."

That afternoon, while sitting in a chair in my living room, holding my almost three week old baby, I experienced pain that I did not know was possible. The pain was so intense that it made the pain from the original two dissections feel like little thumps. It started at the base of the back of my neck, and it ran up into my head. It was a sharp, ripping pain. I thought I was going to lose consciousness as it happened. I yelled for my husband to come take the baby from my arms, and he then helped me to the bed. He called the neurologist, and we were told to go to the ER but not to expect help with the pain. The pain was so severe that my husband called the physician a second time later in the evening and was told the same thing. (If I had it to do all over again, I would have gone to the emergency department).

I sat up all night long in the bed, beside my sleeping husband. I prayed my way through the night. I was afraid to be alone and afraid to go to sleep. Even if I could have slept through the unbearable pain, I was afraid that I would die. The next morning, we were waiting at the neurologist's office when it opened. I insisted on seeing my physician. She called ahead and then sent me to the emergency department, where I was immediately taken back to have an MR-A. My fears were confirmed; I had dissected a third vessel, my right vertebral artery. It was 100% blocked.

  I was admitted into the ICU, uncertain about the reason for the event and what would happen next. The days and weeks that followed were uncertain for me and my family. My husband was at home caring for a newborn and a toddler, and I was medically unstable. After spending my 33rd birthday and two weeks in the hospital, I was released. I was told to try not to sneeze or cough, not to lift anything heavier than a fork, not to drive, and not to make any sudden or unusual head or neck movements. No one could tell me if I would dissect another artery, or why this was happening. We had more questions than we had answers.

  We sought out genetic testing to help figure out why I had dissected 3 cervical arteries. I tested negative for the known genes that cause Ehlers-Danlos

Syndrome (EDS), type IV (the vascular subtype), meaning that I could have an undocumented genetic mutation causing vascular Ehlers-Danlos, or I could have hypermobile type with an undocumented variant, or I could have a connective tissue disorder that closely mimics Ehlers-Danlos but has not been identified yet. I was diagnosed with hypermobile Ehlers-Danlos Syndrome, a connective tissue disorder (think of it as the glue that holds your body together) that affects every system in the body, causing pain, fatigue, joint dislocations, gastrointestinal problems, and a host of other symptoms.

Countless prayers were sent up by family, friends, church, and strangers. People I didn't even know in my community would see me months later, introduce themselves, and tell me that they had been praying for me. Everyone poured kindness out upon us, helping me, caring for our children, driving me to appointments, making meals for us, and just being there for us in general. I will never forget the love and kindness that was shown to us during that time.

As for my dissections, all three were healed at my six month scan, which was much quicker than I expected. I was able to stop Coumadin at that time. I have been advised to remain on Plavix and a beta-blocker for life. I did return to work at the six month mark, after much begging and pleading. Unfortunately, I had to quit working again five years post-dissections, likely permanently this time. My husband, Sidney, has been my hero during all of this, shouldering my slack and never wavering with his love and support.

Early on after my dissections, every time I had a slight pain, I was afraid that another dissection was beginning. For the most part, I've since learned to mostly differentiate when I have to go to the emergency department, although sometimes it is truly difficult to know when to go. I had pulsatile tinnitus for around 6 months after my dissections. The constant, horrible head pain from my vertebral dissection continued for around a year, although we did eventually find a medication that helped some. Today, I continue to have memory difficulties and pains that quickly run up the lines of my vertebral arteries (both of them, even though only one dissected). I have been instructed to lie down during these times in case "another event is about to happen."

To this day, every physician I have seen has said that I could have had a massive stroke and died. None of the them can explain why I didn't. But God has a different plan for my life. If you have survived a dissection and been given another chance at life, I would encourage you to find your purpose. I spent many months trying to figure this out, until I finally realized that it's not just one big purpose that God has for my life, but rather it's a lot of smaller reasons. The reason that I am here today may be different from the reason I was here yesterday. None of us are promised tomorrow.

    I would also encourage you to reach out and find support from others who have experienced similar circumstances. I am so thankful for the internet to be able to connect with survivors all over the world through support groups on Facebook. You are not alone! My last word of advice is if you know something is wrong, do not give up! Be persistent until someone listens. You are your own best advocate!

Husband's Perspective:

    As someone who grew up rarely setting foot in a doctor's office, I was largely unprepared for the course my life was to take in the spring of 2010.

    There have been many highs and lows in our medical odyssey. Early on, I remember mainly the frustration of not knowing what was happening and the long, worried hours of waiting in ERs, hospital rooms, and doctor's offices. As her case is so rare, her doctors – though mostly well-intentioned – were often unable to provide an explanation. Many nurses and doctors were helpful and I am so thankful for them.

I'll never forget feeding our newborn baby in a hospital waiting area as my wife was taken back on a stretcher, or the helpless feeling as I visited her in ICU. Some of the good things I remember are being together as a family at home as she recuperated after the dissections, and a particularly concerned and caring neurologist who was kind and attentive. I am also thankful for the wonderful dissection survivor who spoke with me by phone and gave me hope, and the outpouring of love from family and friends who brought food, sat with our kids, and gave us encouragement.

I love my wife very much, and it's been hard to watch her go through so much. No one wants to see his best friend and life partner suffer. I have watched my wife grow and mature in her faith and in how she reacts to life and meets each hurdle with grace.

Chapter 5:
Diagnostic Tools

"How is a carotid or vertebral artery dissection diagnosed?"

The American Heart Association/American Stroke Association states that there is no one gold standard test that emergency departments should solely depend on, and there are possibilities of false negatives (missing the dissection) with all of the current non-invasive diagnostic tools. Additionally, evidence of an intimal flap, mural hematoma (bleeding in the wall of the artery), stenosis (narrowing), and occlusion do not always appear right away after a dissection.[43]

First and foremost, the level of suspicion for cervical artery dissection must be present. A healthcare professional usually has to be aware that a dissection is a possibility to order the most useful test. For example, in a patient with neck pain, one might order an MRI of the cervical spine (neck), but this test will not provide high-quality images of the carotid and vertebral arteries. There are times when a severe carotid artery dissection near the base of the skull might be visualized on an MRI of the brain, but an MRI of the brain alone will typically miss small dissections, vertebral artery dissections, and carotid dissections lower in the neck.

A radiological study looking specifically at the arteries in the neck should be performed in order to accurately diagnose a carotid or vertebral artery dissection, such as an MR-angiogram (MR-A) or a CT-angiogram (CT-A). Simply put, an MR-angiogram is an MRI study that evaluates the flow of blood within the arteries, rather than focusing on soft tissue or bone. This can be performed either with a contrast ("dye") agent through an IV, or can be done without contrast, although without contrast the quality of the study when evaluating arteries in the neck is variable. A CT-angiogram is a CT scan that is performed after the injection of contrast through an IV to evaluate the flow of the contrast material through the arteries. These radiological tests are imperfect (sensitivities vary), but most studies report relatively good sensitivities with both MR-A and CT-A.

Research studies have found that a CT-A is approximately 90% sensitive in identifying a dissection.[44] If a healthcare provider suspects a carotid or vertebral dissection, CT-A is a preferred diagnostic tool. CT-A is also able to identify features associated with dissection such as intimal flaps, mural hematomas, areas of stenosis, occlusions, and pseudoaneurysms.[45] CT-A is faster and less expensive than an MR-A, and provides high-quality visualization of the carotid and vertebral arteries.[46] The downside to a CT-A is the injection of IV contrast, which has the potential to cause kidney injury (known as contrast nephropathy), particularly in patients who already have kidney disease, as well as exposure to a relatively small amount of radiation. This risk is relatively small, and often the benefit of obtaining an accurate study quickly in a patient experiencing stroke symptoms outweighs this potential risk, but it should still be considered. IV contrast allergies are also not uncommon, so if a patient has a history of an IV contrast allergy, this should also be factored into the decision. If the study is urgently needed and an MR-A is not an option, radiology departments can treat patients with steroids and diphenhydramine ahead of administering a contrast dose to reduce the risk of an allergic reaction.

An MR-A also uses contrast to visualize arteries but does not expose the patient to radiation. An MR-A can visualize arteries without interference from bony segments which is especially useful where vertebral arteries bend around the cervical vertebrae and enter the skull.[47] MR-A can visualize arteries in more detail and find present ischemia but have less accuracy than a CT-A in diagnosing cervical artery dissections. A standard MR-A has approximately 83% sensitivity in diagnosing a carotid artery dissection and only 20% sensitivity in diagnosing a vertebral artery dissection.[48] This is likely due to the vertebral arteries being smaller in size than the carotid arteries and being surrounded by bone (more susceptible to erroneous signals, known as artifact). The new MR-A protocols that use T1 fat saturation sequences, however, are highly sensitive for detecting vertebral and carotid dissection. There are newer high-resolution MR-A diagnostic scans that have promising potential for imaging dissections in vertebral arteries.[49] In one publication, for example, new high-resolution MR-As were able to detect dissections in the extremely sinuous segment of the vertebral artery around C3 (third cervical vertebra) while standard MR-As produced falsely negative results (missed the dissection).[50]

MR-A does not require the use of IV contrast, although the quality of images will likely be higher if IV contrast is used. Contrast for a brain MRI or MR-A is a different substance than IV contrast used for a CT-A. Patients with allergies to IV contrast used in CT scans may tolerate MRI contrast very well, although a small percentage of patients may have allergies to both.

An MRI can be quite long and loud, and some patients feel claustrophobic during the study because the space is somewhat enclosed. If this is a problem for you, "open" MRI scanners are available on a limited basis. Most patients with severe claustrophobia needing to undergo an MRI or an MR-A receive medication to alleviate anxiety, such as diazepam (Valium) or lorazepam (Ativan) before the MRI is performed.

The diagnostic test that provides the most accurate and reliable images of a cervical artery dissection is a digital subtraction angiogram (DSA), also called a catheter arteriogram. Sometimes it is referred to as just an angiogram. Catheter angiography involves placing a catheter (a specialized wire) directly into an artery (usually the femoral artery in the groin region, but the radial artery in the arm has become a popular access point for angiography more recently). The catheter is fed into the artery of interest, such as a carotid or vertebral artery, to deliver contrast into the vessel, and capture up close, real-time images of contrast flowing through it. It is the most sensitive and specific test (the "gold standard") for diagnosing a dissection.

However, placing a catheter into the arterial system is much more invasive than performing an MR-A or a CT-A. It also carries risks that accompany more invasive procedures. In one case series, neurological complications occurred during 2.3% of catheter cerebral angiograms.[51] This number does not include non-neurological complications, such as bleeding at the groin site.

Dissection itself can be a complication of a catheter angiogram. Those with conditions such as fibromuscular dysplasia (FMD) that result in tortuous (twisted) vessels and narrowing throughout the artery may be at an even higher risk for additional dissections resulting from a catheter arteriogram in part because of the challenge of navigating a catheter through these abnormal arteries.

"I thought I didn't have a stroke because my head CT scan was normal, but I did. What happened?"

One of the fastest and least expensive tools for imaging the brain is a computerized tomography (CT) scan. CT scans use x-rays and computer processing to create cross-sectional images (slices) to visualize bones, blood vessels, and soft tissue. Unfortunately, the routine CT scans of the head without contrast will largely miss carotid and vertebral artery dissections, leading to delays in the diagnosis and subsequent stroke or death.[52]

A healthcare provider might assume that a patient with stroke-like symptoms is not having a stroke or a TIA because the head CT scan is normal. *This is flawed reasoning.* The sensitivity of a CT scan without contrast within the first 12-24 hours of an ischemic stroke is around 65%, meaning that 35% of patients presenting 12-24 hours after a stroke has started will have essentially normal head CT scans. The sensitivity is much lower for patients presenting to the emergency department within several hours of a stroke or stroke-like symptoms.

A head CT scan is a very good tool for diagnosing bleeding that occurs in the brain, and this is the reason why patients presenting with stroke symptoms are supposed to have a CT scan – *to look for blood* (a hemorrhagic stroke). The purpose of a CT scan should not be to diagnose or rule out an ischemic stroke. The likelihood of detecting hemorrhage in the brain is around 90-95% with a CT scan, but a CT scan should never be used to "rule out" stroke within the first day after stroke-like symptoms develop.

"What is the difference between a CT scan and an MRI?"

The simple answer is that a CT scan uses x-rays to construct images, whereas MRI uses a magnetic field to create images. The technologies behind both are more complex than this would suggest though.

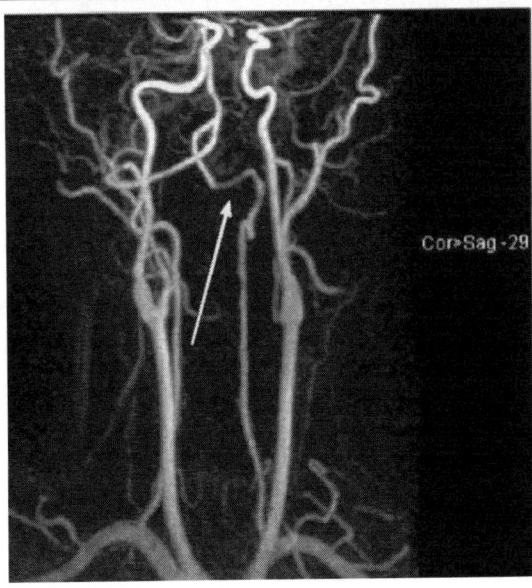

Figure 13[53]
The MR-A featured demonstrates evidence of a left vertebral artery dissection (arrow). There is narrowing and irregularity in the artery, but it is not occluded.

From a practical standpoint, CT scans generally take less time to complete than MRI studies. When a patient first arrives in the emergency department with signs and symptoms concerning for stroke, a CT scan of the head is a *quick* way to effectively rule out bleeding in the brain. However, as was stated in the previous section, a CT scan does *not* rule out an ischemic stroke.

A brain MRI is a much more sensitive radiological study for detecting early ischemia in the brain. Some hospitals have built protocols around getting a few key sets of images quickly in patients with stroke-like symptoms to guide management in the emergency department. However, for most hospitals getting a brain MRI is more time-consuming, and when every minute counts (as it does with stroke), the CT is preferred because it can be completed within a few short minutes.

"What are some other diagnostic tools that can be used to diagnose a cervical artery dissection?"

Duplex ultrasound can also be used to diagnose a cervical artery dissection. A carotid ultrasound is a non-invasive imaging tool that evaluates blood flow in the arteries of the neck, and does not expose the patient to radiation or contrast. Duplex ultrasonography measures the velocity (essentially, the speed) at which blood is flowing in an artery, and can detect occlusion or significant stenosis. Depending on the degree of arterial stenosis, duplex ultrasound is not as precise as other imaging techniques, and cannot determine if a patient has had a stroke. If the artery has only narrowed slightly, the ability of the test to find a dissection drops as low as 40%.[54] However, if an artery is completely occluded, the sensitivity of the test is as high as 100%.

It is not always possible to distinguish between stenosis caused by atherosclerosis and dissection.

Additionally, only sections of the internal carotid arteries in the neck can be evaluated, because once the arteries pass the jaw, there are no bone "windows" for detecting flow through the vessels until the carotid siphon (segment near the eye).

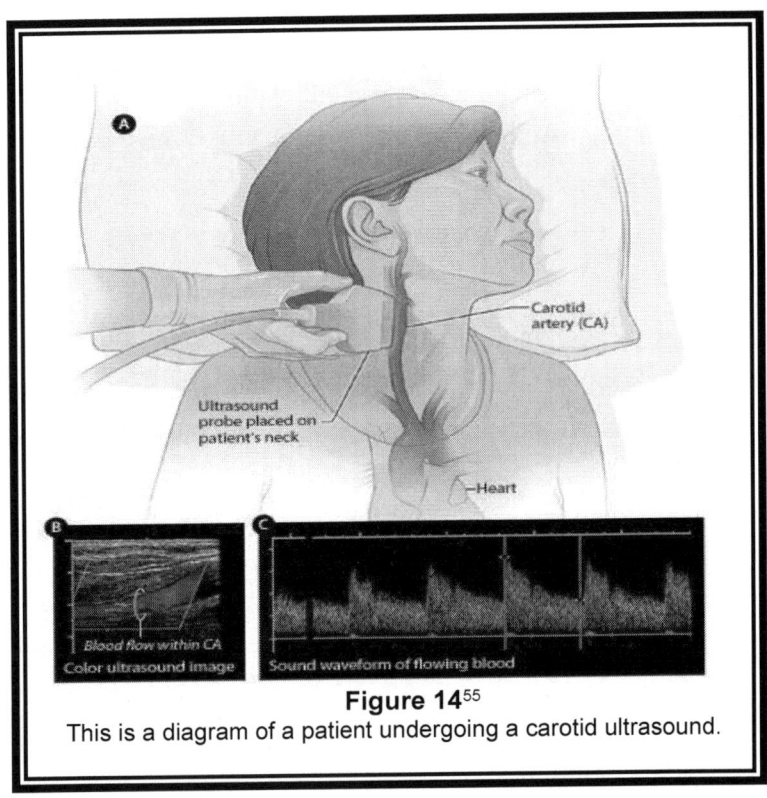

Figure 14[55]
This is a diagram of a patient undergoing a carotid ultrasound.

Below are some ultrasound images of a dissection flap in a carotid artery. The first image is a head-on cross-section (axial section) of a dissected carotid artery, while the second image is a side view cross-section (sagittal section). An arrow points to the flap.

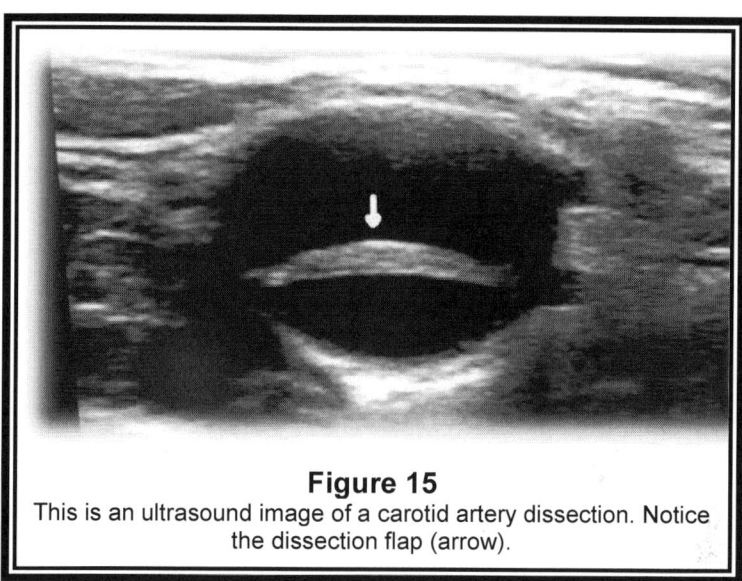

Figure 15
This is an ultrasound image of a carotid artery dissection. Notice the dissection flap (arrow).

These are exceptionally clear images, and not all ultrasounds of the cervical arteries show dissections so clearly. The American Stroke Association recommends using non-invasive testing and cautions providers not to rely on a single test for diagnostic purposes.[56]

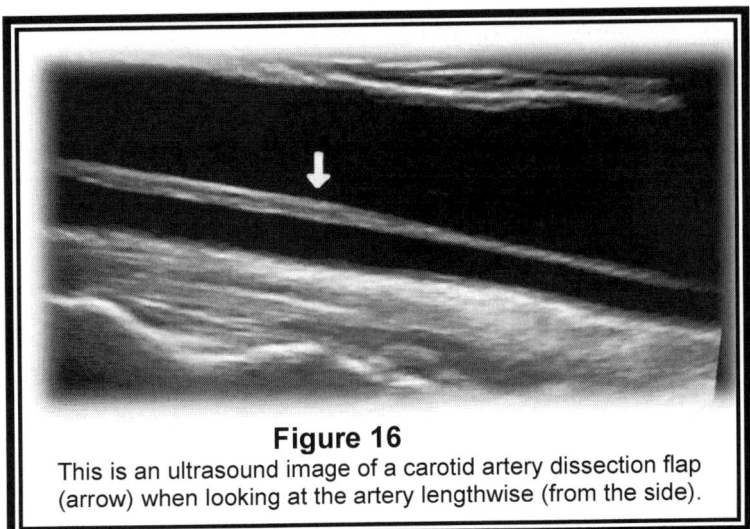

Figure 16
This is an ultrasound image of a carotid artery dissection flap (arrow) when looking at the artery lengthwise (from the side).

"I just had a carotid ultrasound performed, and the report says that I have '0-50%' narrowing in my artery. Why doesn't it tell me exactly how narrow it is?"

In a carotid ultrasound study, the interpreter estimates the degree of narrowing in an artery by measuring the velocity, or speed, at which blood is flowing at various sites along the artery. Because the results are based on an approximate calculation, you will only receive a range of narrowing, such as "less than 50% narrowing," "50-69% narrowing," or "70-99% stenosis."

"On the MR-A of my neck, the report just said that my vertebral artery was 'not well-visualized' but that dissection could not be ruled out. What does that mean?"

If there is no blood flow in an artery, the blood vessel will not be visible in that segment because there is no contrast reaching that part of the artery to show up on the MRI. Even if the MR-A is performed without contrast, depending on the angle of the artery, flow may be difficult to see in particular segments.

Sometimes a blood vessel may be poorly visualized simply because the patient moved during the test, or the vessel itself may be hypoplastic (undeveloped). Occasionally, the MRI picks up images of areas around the blood vessel but misses the vessel itself. In addition to these MR-A limitations, a vessel may also be hard to see on a CT-A if the timing of the IV contrast injection is not coordinated well with the scan, since the contrast may not have arrived in the artery yet when the pictures are taken. If there is question about a diagnosis, but a high suspicion for dissection, another vascular imaging study should be performed.

"I thought my MR-A looked pretty abnormal, but my neurologist said there was only 'motion artifact.' What does that mean?"

Movement during an MRI can cause distortion in the image. Unfortunately, this distortion can result from even the slightest of motions, such as those required for breathing. Even your pulse throughout your artery can result in some distortion of the image. Since the cervical arteries contract with each heartbeat it is impossible to stop this type of movement, no matter how still you try to lie. A radiologist, neurologist, or neurosurgeon can usually determine what findings result from movement and what could be a concerning vascular abnormality.

"When should healthcare providers perform an MR-angiogram or a CT-angiogram to look for a cervical artery dissection?"

Any time patients present with traditional stroke-like symptoms (weakness on one side, numbness on one side, facial droop, slurred speech, difficulty with word finding, trouble swallowing, etc.) and a head CT does not show evidence of bleeding in the brain, an imaging study of the vessels in the neck should be performed to better understand what could be causing these symptoms. However, a relatively young patient lacking stroke-like symptoms who presents with a severe headache and/or neck pain without any similar history of such presentation should have an MR-A or a CT-A to exclude cervical artery dissection.

Intense head and neck pain are crucial warning signs before the onset of stroke in patients with both vertebral and carotid artery dissections.[57] If a patient presents with a combination of head and neck pain, Horner syndrome, pulsatile tinnitus, and/or taste and visual disturbances, suspicion for a carotid dissection should be high, and an MR-A or CT-A should be pursued to confirm or rule out the diagnosis.[58]

"How often should I get a scan of my dissected artery? Should I keep getting follow-up scans even after my artery has healed?"

If you are a patient who has had a carotid or vertebral artery dissection, and you frequently wish you could undergo repeated CT-As or MR-As just to check on your artery, please know that this is a very normal feeling. It is common to feel anxiety over the current status of your artery and to want to know if your artery is healing properly. Following a dissection, patients often worry over whether another dissection could occur.

There is no standard guideline about repeat imaging after carotid or vertebral artery dissection. Many neurologists will repeat a CT-A or an MR-A anywhere eeks to six months following the dissection to t the dissection is resolving and to provide ...ance about the particular medical therapy the patient is taking. For example, if a patient is on an anticoagulation drug like warfarin, the risk of hemorrhaging as an adverse effect will be higher compared to a patient who is on aspirin daily. Seeing evidence of a healed dissection with good flow through the artery may persuade a neurologist to stop anticoagulation drugs and start aspirin in its place. Another physician may have a patient on aspirin, and if the vessel looks normal on repeat imaging, he or she may recommend discontinuing the aspirin altogether.

If you are feeling confused about the lack of consensus on how to manage cervical artery dissections after the acute event, it is because there is a serious lack of evidence guiding providers in how to provide care.

Most agree that if a patient with a history of a cervical artery dissection presents with new/recurrent severe neck pain, another intense headache similar to the one that was present at the time of the dissection, or other new neurological symptoms that could be consistent with TIA or stroke, that ordering a repeat CT-A or MR-A is justified.

Often patients will want repeat scans beyond the six month time frame "just to check on things." Please know that we understand this desire and empathize. A patient told us once: "If I could get a scan every week I would do it." Enduring a dissection and its aftermath is an anxiety-provoking experience. Unfortunately, this is usually not feasible without new symptoms. Insurers may not be willing to approve such neuroimaging studies without a new indication (new symptoms). Remember as well that, even though the risk with CT-As and MR-As is relatively low, there are always risks associated with any procedure.

In the United States, there is very wide range of prices for diagnostic tests. What you may not realize is that you have a choice regarding where you can get your scan if this test is being performed in the outpatient setting. A few minutes of calling diagnostic centers and getting quotes for MR-As and CT-As can save you hundreds (possibly thousands, depending on the test) of dollars. It is also worthwhile to understand whether your insurance will cover non-urgent CT-As or MR-As at only particular facilities in your region, so that you do not find yourself with a hefty bill from having used an imaging center outside of your network.

Chapter 6: Patient Story
The Adjustment

I was 32 years old when, I suffered a left vertebral artery dissection at C1 with an occipital stroke within an hour after a chiropractic cervical manipulation. I had been seeing a chiropractor for around two years prior to this visit at the recommendation of a TMJ specialist to address my jaw pain. This particular visit was for the jaw pain as well as some minor neck pain I had been experiencing for about a week after a brief stomach virus. This was my first visit to this particular chiropractor and my first chiropractic visit overall in at least 3 months.

My appointment was on September 10. The chiropractor manipulated my back, hips, and neck with her hands, and then she used an actuator on my jaw. I was out of the office in less than 15 minutes and driving to pick up my son from daycare when I started seeing white spots in both eyes. The spots were small, like spots that remain briefly after a camera flash, but they would not go away. I wear contacts, so I remember checking my eyes in the mirror and rubbing them, thinking something was on my contacts. The spots continued.

After picking up my son from daycare, on the drive home, I noticed I had no peripheral vision. Within the hour, my husband was cooking dinner, and I was sitting on the floor in our den nursing my son when I became dizzy and felt faint. I called my husband into the room because I felt like I might drop my son. When my husband ran in, I could not see him. He sat on the floor directly in front of me, but I could only see portions of his face. I recall rubbing my eyes and saying that I felt like my eyes were doing weird things. He responded that my eyes were moving all around, in different directions from each other. This lasted for only moments, and then I felt an intense warm rush up the back of my neck.

After the rush sensation stopped, my vision went back to normal. I could see with no spots. There was no dizziness, and my strength felt normal. Then suddenly the most intense headache I have ever had hit me. I had no idea that I had just experienced a stroke. That honestly never crossed my mind. I did feel that whatever was happening was related to the chiropractic visit. The chiropractor's office was still open, so I called and told the receptionist what happened. She told me that the chiropractor would be at my house within 15 minutes, and she was.

When the chiropractor arrived at my house, she checked my blood pressure and used the flashlight on my smartphone to check my pupils. She never mentioned a stroke. She explained to me that what I experienced could have been because I was dehydrated from nursing or that my nerves were overly sensitive because it had been a few months since an adjustment. She also mentioned she could have over-rotated something. She did a few pressure point presses for my headache and told me to go to the ER if it happened again.

My headache continued for two days, but I was otherwise normal. On the following day, September 11, I was examined by an orthopedic specialist, thinking that what I had experienced was a ruptured disc or something related to my spine. He took x-rays of my cervical spine with normal results. He said I had less curvature in my neck than normal but explained that was typical of someone with a sore neck and that it would return to normal once I felt better.

I explained to him what happened the night before after leaving the chiropractor. He told me that I had "dodged a bullet," and told me a terrible story about his friend's wife who had a dissection and stroke after a chiropractic visit, and she had to have permanent help as a result. He said that I was "out of the woods for anything like that" because I was feeling normal. He referred me for physical therapy for what he described as some inflammation in my neck. I remember calling my husband as I drove back to my office and crying as I told him the story about the doctor's friend. I remember crying because it was such a scary story and because I was so shocked that something like that could happen. I vividly remember driving and talking about how grateful I was that that had not happened to me!

  On September 12, I woke up with no headache. I'm an attorney, and that morning I had a court appearance and a couple of in-office meetings in the afternoon. The morning was fine, and I recall feeling more like myself, but around 3 P.M. I started seeing white spots again while sitting at my desk. One of the partners at my law firm walked into my office about the same time and said my eyes were moving in opposite directions. A co-worker took me to the ER. There, I waited for over two hours to be seen because they treated me as though I only had a migraine. I was finally seen by the ER doctor, who ordered a CT scan. The radiologist said it did not show anything; however, the ER doctor was not satisfied. Luckily for me, the ER doctor remembered several artery dissections he had previously seen. According to my nurse, the ER doctor had a heated discussion with the radiologist and explained that I was "not fabricating my symptoms" and "something was really wrong." He said I was not leaving until they found out what was happening. He ordered a CT- angiogram, MRI of the cervical spine, and an MRI of the brain with and without contrast. With these tests, they found my dissection and a spot on the back, right side of my brain possibly from the stroke. After consulting with the neurologist on call, I was given an aspirin and discharged home at 2 A.M. with an appointment with a neurologist the following morning.

    When I arrived at the neurologist's office, he was already familiar with my situation. He explained that the spot on the back, right side of my brain was a stroke. He said that would explain the vision problems. He told me to make arrangements for my son and then to return to the hospital to be admitted. He explained he wanted me to have a repeat CT-angiogram and to get started on blood thinners in the hospital, where I could be monitored due to the risk of another stroke when the blood thinners were started. I was in the hospital for the weekend (September 13-15). I was on baby aspirin during this time and had a repeat CT-angiogram and MRIs. The two neurologists treating me during this time were not certain about a treatment plan. They brought me one option for medications, then changed the recommendation after they consulted with a "stroke expert" and a radiologist. Ultimately, we decided I would remain on baby aspirin and add gabapentin and Plavix. On Sunday, I was discharged home, with the medications but no physical restrictions. (During this hospital visit, I was not able to nurse my son due to the dye from the scans. Then, I had to give up nursing completely due to the medications prescribed.)

During the following week, I had very low energy. I finally felt well enough to get dressed and leave the house on September 19. After running errands, I was driving on the interstate back home when I had a sharp pain shoot up the left side of my head and simultaneous double vision for a split second. My car swerved a little but not out of my lane. I had a friend take me back to the emergency room, where, fortunately, the same ER doctor was working. He told me that I had experienced a TIA. New scans were taken, but they did not show any changes, so my neurologists did not want to change my treatment plan. A doctor friend of mine came up to the ER to check on me and spoke with the ER doctor; both he and my friend disagreed with the neurologists. My friend contacted a neurosurgeon, and the neurosurgeon took over my care moving forward.

With the neurosurgeon involved, I was transferred by ambulance to a university hospital. I was admitted and underwent a catheter arteriogram (through the groin) the following morning (September 20). During the catheter arteriogram, I learned that genetically I only have one functioning vertebral artery, the left. The right vertebral artery is present, but is smaller and does not reach the Circle of Willis. The neurosurgeon said the left vertebral artery was 65% occluded. He placed me on Coumadin and said I would be okay in 3-6 months. He also placed me under physical restrictions, specifically nothing that would strain my neck. No exercise, no running, no swift head movements, no extreme motion of the head, no driving, and no lifting or carrying anything 25 pounds or more, which was particularly devastating for me because it meant I could not pick up my son.

    I remained in the hospital through the weekend. I was instructed to give myself Lovenox injections until I became therapeutic on Coumadin. I gave myself my first injection on Saturday night. I was discharged on September 22, with Lovenox injections twice a day and a referral for a primary care physician to manage my Coumadin.

    I had a follow up appointment with the neurosurgeon on September 24. I could barely walk by that time. The neurosurgeon ordered an ultrasound and found that I had developed a pseudoaneurysm in my leg from the angiogram. I was admitted back into the hospital again. I was scheduled for surgery the following morning for the pseudoaneurysm; however, I became violently ill, and the surgery was postponed. Turns out, during the hospital stays, I contracted *Clostridium difficile* ("C. diff"), an infection of the colon. With my surgery postponed, a second ultrasound of my leg was ordered, and it was found that the pseudoaneurysm had healed on its own. I was then treated for the C. diff., and became therapeutic on Coumadin during the hospital stay. I was discharged on September 27, on Coumadin along with nausea medication and Flagyl for the C. diff.

    At the time of my dissection, I was a full-time associate attorney with a prominent law firm, a wife, and mother to a seven month old baby. Because of the dissection, I had severe headaches while looking at a computer screen so I was off work without pay from September 23 through January 16, when I finally felt well enough to return. When I returned, I was only comfortable performing office work. I did not travel for court or depositions because I was not supposed to be driving, and also because my symptoms increased if my blood pressure changed even slightly.

    The symptoms I experienced while my artery was dissected were mostly dizziness and fatigue. For months, I had the feeling like I had just stepped off a boat. I also still have pain at the spot of the dissection. The neurosurgeon told me most of his vertebral artery dissection patients report head and neck pain. He said that would be my new normal. My experience has been that I will have dizziness and pain with almost every activity I do post-dissection, but once I continue to do the activity for weeks, the dizziness and pain stops occurring. For example, when the dissection occurred, I could not unload the dishwasher without having to go lie down for several hours. After a few weeks, though, I was able to unload the dishwasher like normal again; however, this activity did result in trips to the ER.

  With my dissection in the left vertebral artery, and my anatomical variant of only having one functioning artery, the neurosurgeon explained that should my left artery completely occlude, that would be the "end of the ballgame" for me, or, at the very least, put me at risk for another stroke. He said that the only way for me to know that my condition is worsening is if my symptoms increase. With that, anytime I experienced what seemed like an increase in symptoms, I went to the ER. Thankfully, my artery had healed itself after 6 months. The neurosurgeon performed another angiogram on March 27 to confirm the healing shown on the scans. The angiogram confirmed the dissection was healed, and the stenosis completely cleared up. I remain on baby aspirin indefinitely now.

(Note: This is one patient's personal story, and the care plan described is not endorsed by the authors of this book. Catheter angiography as a procedure carries a 1-2% risk of stroke and a risk of vascular injury at the catheter access point, and less invasive methods of imaging arteries for this purpose, such as CT-A or MR-A, are usually adequate for confirming dissection healing.)

Chapter 7:
Causes

"What causes carotid and vertebral artery dissections?"

This is possibly the most common question that neurologists receive from patients with cervical artery dissections. The typical reaction from a patient after an initial diagnosis of a carotid or vertebral artery dissection is one of shock because this vascular injury was nowhere on his or her radar.

In a healthy person without any known predisposition for weakness within the walls of his or her arteries, direct trauma to the neck can cause what is known as a traumatic dissection. Sudden severe extension of the neck, or "whiplash," such as from a motor vehicle collision, is a common cause of traumatic dissection.

Other activities that have been associated with cervical artery dissections include:
- Neck "adjustments," more formally referred to as cervical manipulations
- Prolonged coughing
- Sneezing
- Straining to lift a heavy load

- Neck extension during hair wash at a salon (also called the "beauty parlor dissection")
- Swimming (turning the head quickly to the side)
- Intense yelling
- Vomiting
- Sudden neck extension or jerking neck movement (such as on a roller coaster)
- Extreme (or sometimes even not-so-extreme) exercise or stretching

These may also be considered "traumatic" dissections, because there is a specific inciting physical factor associated with it. Some may argue that since these are all relatively normal activities, they should not result in such a dramatic vascular injury and there may be an underlying unknown connective tissue disorder which may have caused the injury. Activities do not have to involve direct trauma to result in cervical artery dissection. An abrupt increase in pressure within the artery in combination with stress or strain to the arterial wall can occur during activities thought to be harmless. Remember from our first Patient Story that Amanda dissected her carotid artery while trying to blow up a balloon.

The unfortunate reality as well is that nearly half of patients with carotid or vertebral artery dissection will have no idea what caused it. Symptoms will emerge, but there is no specific moment when a patient realizes something is wrong. He or she may awaken in the morning with a headache, or abruptly develop TIA or stroke symptoms with a baseline neck ache or mild headache, only to be diagnosed with the dissection as part of the evaluation for the neurological deficits. These are known as spontaneous dissections.

"I thought I was a healthy person. However, since my dissection, I have now been diagnosed with fibromuscular dysplasia. What is that?"

About five percent of cervical artery dissections are caused by identifiable underlying vascular and/or genetic abnormalities. Fibromuscular dysplasia, FMD, is a disorder that results in abnormal cellular development in one or more arterial walls. FMD is a relatively rare disease. According to the American Stroke Association, there are currently 921 cases in the United States that have been identified in a national registry. However, the condition is very likely underdiagnosed. About 20% of these registry patients have had an arterial dissection either in their carotid, vertebral, or renal arteries (arteries carrying blood to the kidneys).[59]

The arterial walls of individuals with FMD are susceptible to narrowing (stenosis), aneurysms, and dissections. FMD may cause an artery to appear like a "string of beads" with kinks and bulges, but other conditions can mimic this appearance on CT-As, MR-As, and catheter angiography images.

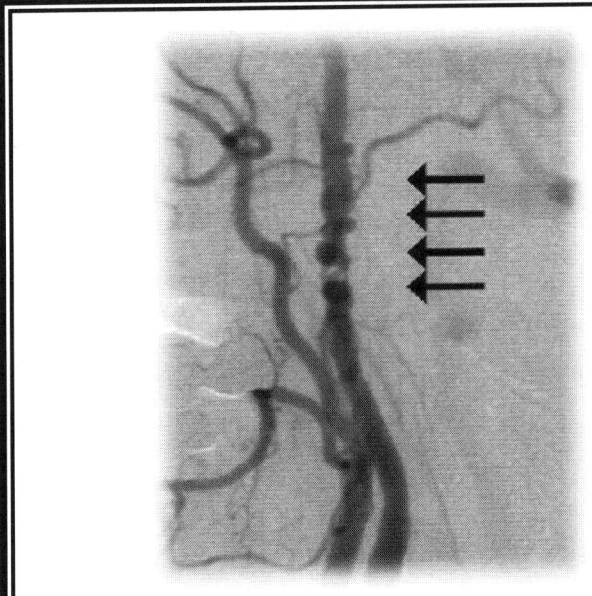

Figure 17[60]
The image illustrates the "string of beads" formation in a carotid artery, characteristic of FMD.

FMD is more common among women, comprising over 90% of the FMD population in one study.[61] It is typically diagnosed in patients approximately 30-50 years of age and is believed to stem from genetic abnormalities.[62] Carotid artery dissections are more common in patients with FMD than vertebral artery dissections.[63] Typically, FMD is diagnosed after a health problem such as a stroke, and it is discovered during diagnostic imaging tests.

"Now that I have been diagnosed with FMD, is there anything else I should do?"

The American College of Cardiology Foundation recommends that patients diagnosed with FMD receive "one-time cross-sectional imaging from head to pelvis with computed tomographic angiography or magnetic resonance angiography."[64] People with FMD have a higher risk for dissection and aneurysms, and a diagnostic test can help identify potentially dangerous vascular abnormalities that may require medical intervention.

"I have always been 'double-jointed' but didn't think much about it. My doctor thinks I have Ehlers-Danlos syndrome and that it contributed to my dissection. What is that?"

Ehlers-Danlos syndrome (EDS) is a group of inherited disorders that impairs the integrity of connective tissue. Blood vessel walls, joints, and skin have excessive elasticity, making individuals susceptible to cervical artery dissections.

Most sources estimate the prevalence of EDS globally to be about 1 in 5,000 individuals. However, most cases of EDS thought to be correlated with vascular dissections occur in people with EDS, type IV. There are multiple forms of EDS, but type IV is known as "vascular" EDS, which is due to a genetic mutation in the COL3A gene that results in abnormal synthesis of type-III collagen. Patients with EDS, type IV, frequently develop life-threatening complications at relatively young ages, either due to dissection, aneurysm rupture and hemorrhaging, or frank organ rupture. EDS, type IV is a relatively rare disorder, affecting about 1 in 50,000 to 1 in 200,000 people.[65]

Individuals with EDS present with overly flexible joints. Smaller joints in the hands and arms are particularly flexible (Figure 18). Individuals may also have stretchy and fragile skin that bruises and tears easily. Facial features include a thin nose, thin upper lip, prominent eyes, and small earlobes. These patients may also be able to touch the tips of their tongues to the tip of their noses. EDS can cause translucent skin with visible veins and arteries in particularly fair individuals.

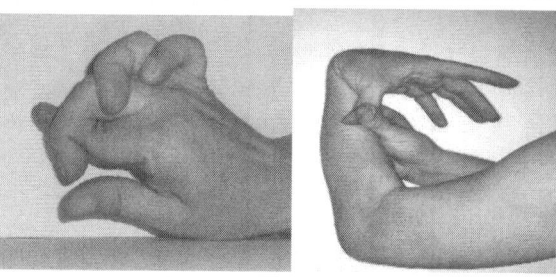

Figure 18[66]
These two photographs depict the overly flexible joints of the hands a characteristic of Ehlers-Danlos syndrome.

Genetic testing is available for COL3A mutations if there is concern for EDS, type IV, following a dissection. Genetic panels also exist for the most common mutations resulting in the various types of EDS. If you are interested in learning more about genetic testing, GeneTests® is a website that provides a thorough overview of the of genetic tests available (http://www.genetests.org).

"I was reading online about a condition called Marfan syndrome that can cause dissections. What is that?"

Marfan syndrome is a genetic disorder that results in less robust connective tissue due to a mutation in the fibrillin gene. Individuals with Marfan syndrome typically have the following features:

- Tall stature
- Long legs, arms, and fingers
- Spine curvature
- Concave or protruding rib cage
- Overly flexible joints
- Flat feet
- Crowded teeth
- Stretch marks unrelated to weight gain or loss[67]

Individuals with Marfan syndrome may have potentially life-threatening complications, such as abnormal heart valves and aortic dissections. People with Marfan syndrome may experience sudden lung collapse due to ineffective connective tissue that should keep the lungs attached to the rib cage. Visual impairments such as severe near-sightedness, dislocated lenses, detached retinas, premature cataracts, and glaucoma may also occur.

If you suspect you might have Marfan syndrome, share your concerns with your healthcare provider. The Marfan Foundation has some excellent resources and information for individuals and family members affected by Marfan syndrome.

"I have had a bunch of bone fractures, and after my vertebral artery dissection I read about a condition called osteogenesis imperfecta that can cause fractures and dissections. What is that?"

Osteogenesis imperfecta is a genetic disorder that results in reduced collagen formation, which is a essential to healthy connective tissue that results in extremely brittle bones. A person with osteogenesis imperfecta may have several hundred bone fractures over the course of his or her lifetime.[68] Physical abuse may be suspected in infants and children because of the numerous, recurrent bone fractures, even though abuse is not occurring.

Osteogenesis imperfecta can also lead to dissections of arterial linings, including spontaneous carotid and vertebral dissections. Typically, though, a diagnosis of osteogenesis imperfecta will have been made long before a cervical artery dissection occurs.

"Are there other genetic disorders that can cause carotid and vertebral artery dissections?"

There are a number of other rarer disorders that have been associated with increased risk of carotid and vertebral artery dissection. Loey-Dietz syndrome, for example, arises from a mutation in the TGFBR2 gene, resulting in many features similar to Marfan syndrome.

For further reading about rare genetic disorders, we recommend visiting the Online Mendelian Inheritance in Man (OMIM) website (http://www.omim.org) and searching for "dissection." You will find a wealth of information about these disorders.

"Should I be tested for genetic connective tissue disorders if I have had a dissection?"

Genetic testing is very expensive, and insurers typically request justification for ordering them. Selecting the correct genetic tests is not only based on the presence of a carotid or vertebral dissection, but should also consider the patient's family history, physical and neurological exam, and physical appearance. For example, if a patient with a spontaneous dissection has a textbook appearance of someone with Marfan syndrome, it may make sense to send the FBN1 test (fibrillin 1) to evaluate for Marfan syndrome, and if positive, it will have been worthwhile not to send for a large array of genetic tests that may result in $50,000 in costs. If a patient has incidental aneurysms identified on a CT-A or MR-A, joint flexibility, very prominent eyes, and skin that tears easily, it makes more sense to send a panel evaluating for Ehlers-Danlos syndrome, type IV.

Frequently, it is the case where a patient will have multiple spontaneously dissected arteries, and a wide array of genetic tests have been normal. Why? One possibility is that some patients may be genetically predisposed to some degree of weakness within the arterial wall, but our medical tests are only able to identify what we know to exist at this point in time. Patients with spontaneous cervical artery dissections frequently express frustration over the lack of a specific underlying diagnosis. This frustration can stem from fear and a sense of vulnerability. If the "cause" is unknown, it is difficult to cope with the situation.

    While the known presence of a genetic disorder often leads to more meticulous screening, the reality is that there is no cure at this point for Ehler-Danlos syndrome, Marfan syndrome, osteogenesis imperfecta, or many of the other rarer disorders that can place patients at risk for cervical artery dissections. Given this fact, some question whether genetic testing is worthwhile. Perhaps it is. Some patients think they will find peace of mind with an answer in the form of a positive genetic test. However, it is worth considering that a positive genetic test result for a condition with no cure may create additional anxiety. Some patients find it helpful to talk with a genetics counselor to better understand the pros and cons of genetic testing before proceeding.

"How do I know which precautions to take to avoid another dissection if I don't know what caused it in the first place?"

When patients have multiple spontaneous cervical artery dissections, whether there is a positive genetic test or not, a specific underlying diagnosis or not, they should be treated similarly to those who do have a confirmed diagnosis of a collagen vascular or connective tissue disease. Patients should be cautious with or avoid heavy lifting and straining. Activities resulting in potentially traumatic injuries to the neck should be avoided. Just because genetic testing was negative in a patient with four spontaneous cervical artery dissections, does that mean he or she should return to aggressively boxing? No, it does not.

"I was taking birth control pills at the time of my dissection. Could this have contributed to my dissection and stroke?"

There has been some evidence that birth control pills, migraines, and smoking are associated with an increased risk of cervical artery dissection.[69] The American Heart Association states: "Women who take even a low-estrogen birth control pill may be twice as likely to have a stroke as those who don't and the risk may increase if other risk factors are present."[70] Many oral contraceptive pills contain the hormones estrogen and progesterone, and supplemental estrogen can increase the body's production of blood clots. About one in 3,000 women who are taking birth control pills will develop a blood clot while on them.[71]

Birth control pills have not been shown to directly cause dissections, but they can increase the risk of stroke, especially if an individual possesses additional risk factors. Discuss with your doctor your options for birth control once you have had a dissection.

"My stroke symptoms started after a chiropractor adjusted my neck. Can neck manipulation cause cervical artery dissections?"

This question has been an area of controversy for decades, and patients ask it frequently. In 2014, the American Heart Association (AHA) released a scientific statement reviewing the published evidence on the statistical association between cervical artery dissections and cervical manipulative therapy ("neck adjustment"). The current amount of published evidence was deemed to be insufficient to make a statement that cervical manipulative therapy directly causes cervical artery dissections. However, the group concluded: "...most population controlled studies have found an association between [cervical manipulative therapy] and [vertebral artery dissection] stroke in young patients."[72]

Patients with bilateral vertebral artery dissections have a significantly higher rate of association with chiropractic cervical manipulation.[73] The forceful neck manipulation on both sides resulting in bilateral vertebral artery dissections points to a direct relationship between cervical manipulation and vertebral artery dissection.[74] Cervical manipulation places a shearing force systematically on both vertebral arteries, which is more likely to result in bilateral vertebral artery dissections, in contrast with physical exercise where abrupt movement is more likely to be confined to one side, resulting in only one vertebral dissection.[75]

Spontaneous bilateral vertebral artery dissections in healthy young adults with the absence of a connective tissue disorder are typically rare but occur more often in individuals after chiropractic neck manipulation.

Complications associated with cervical manipulation have been reported since 1947 when Pratt-Thomas and Berger reported two patients who became unconscious during chiropractic manipulation and died within 24 hours after the adjustment.[76] Since 1947, case reports have continued to record vertebral and carotid dissections, stroke and cases of death closely associated with cervical manipulation. A study conducted from 1978 to 1988 in Denmark examining the link between stroke and chiropractic cervical manipulations concluded: "There seems to be sufficient evidence to justify a firm policy statement cautioning against upper cervical rotation."[77]

A 2010 clinical study found 34 cases of death associated with cervical artery dissections after chiropractic manipulation, and a 2013 study of cases between 2001 and 2011 found 707 incidents of stroke after cervical manipulation.[78] One source estimates that 1 in 20,000 cervical spinal manipulations result in a vertebral artery dissection and/or aneurysm.[79] Presentation of neurological symptoms can be up to two months after the initial dissection, but 63% of patients develop symptoms immediately following cervical manipulation.[80]

In response to the AHA's statement, the American Chiropractic Association (ACA) issued a comment, claiming that the AHA statement "fails to show that neck manipulation is a significant risk factor in [cervical arterial dissection]."[81] The ACA comment also claimed that the risk of death from spine surgery was 1,800 per one million people, the risk of death from combined use of nonsteroidal anti-inflammatory drugs (NSAIDs) and aspirin was 153 per one million people, but that the association between neck manipulation and stroke was less than one per one million people.

It is possible that some patients seek cervical manipulation due to neck pain after they have already have dissected an artery. In fact, the ACA has asserted this in defense of cervical manipulation. Chiropractors can be on the front lines of helping patients with early cervical artery dissections, since some of these patients seek their help for relief from the neck pain they are experiencing. Therefore, they can take a proactive role regarding carotid and vertebral dissections if they can be identified clinically by these providers.

Cervical manipulation may worsen an underlying dissection if it was already present. It is possible that some dissections closely associated with chiropractic cervical manipulations represent aggravation of a preexisting dissection, especially if the patient sought help from a chiropractor for new unexplained neck pain. However, the force from a cervical manipulation can put extreme pressure on vertebral and even carotid arteries.

If chiropractors suspect that a patient's neck pain may be due to an acute cervical artery dissection, then they should avoid neck manipulation in the interest of safety.[82] We also assert that patients undergoing cervical manipulation should be informed of the association between this procedure and cervical artery dissection prior to neck adjustment.

"About a week before I was diagnosed with my vertebral dissection I had a cold with a pretty bad cough. Is it possible that coughing caused my dissection?"

Acute respiratory infection has been associated in multiple case series with increased risk of dissection. Some studies have linked respiratory infections to dissections with a seasonal peak in the fall and winter.[83] It is unclear if the dissection is caused from mechanical stresses, such as coughing, or from the systemic effects of the infection itself (or both).[84]

"I've gone over it in my mind again and again, but I can't think of a single thing that could have caused my dissection. How could such a drastic vascular injury occur without any obvious cause?"

Spontaneous cervical artery dissections also occur in individuals without any known connective tissue disorders. Some individuals have no idea what could have triggered their dissections or when they happened because of the delay in the presentation of symptoms. Research indicates that up to 35% of patients have spontaneous dissections without any identified cause.[85]

However, because the actual event that triggered the dissection could be seemingly innocuous, people may be unaware of when the dissection occurred.

Everyday activities have been known to cause the lining of both vertebral and carotid arteries to tear. Since these events do not typically cause dissection in the general population, they are still considered spontaneous dissections. Some researchers have classified them as "mild trauma" or "provoked spontaneous dissection."[86]

These are activities that usually do not lead to severe vascular trauma. The following daily events have been reported to be the aggravating factors in at least one reported case of cervical artery dissection:

Reported Causes of Cervical Dissection

running	biking
aerobics	sneezing
hiking	bowling
child birth	weight lifting
head banging (dance)	basketball
dental procedure	golf
tennis	vomiting
cupping	horseback riding
star gazing	anesthesia
vision exam	gymnastics
yelling	tai chi
waterslide	sleeping position
yoga	nose blowing
massage	coughing
archery	dancing
sex	trampoline
scuba diving	talking on the phone
roller coaster	ceiling painting
swimming	skiing

Many of the activities involve either exercising, stretching, or lifting. When somebody strains to lift an object, the vocal folds adduct (close). We hold our breath when we lift heavy objects, and a group of muscles in the neck contract. The digastric and stylohyoid muscles contract during heavy lifting and run deep into the carotid triangle, where they intertwine with connecting tissue on the lining of the internal carotid artery. Straining and lifting can cause a sudden increase in arterial pressure and can theoretically result in a dissection of the arterial wall.[87]

Place two fingers above your hyoid bone (Adam's apple) and swallow. You will be able to feel the muscles in your neck contract to raise the hyoid bone to initiate a swallow. These muscles also contract during lifting, coughing, straining, and bearing down for childbirth. Excessive force when contracting these muscles could put strain on the lining of the carotid artery and result in a dissection, and you may not realize this when it occurs.

Researchers believe there may be an underlying cause for dissection due to seemingly harmless activity. Some studies have demonstrated that up to 65% of subjects with spontaneous vertebral dissections had multiple dissections present at the same time, pointing to a possible underlying condition that made their arteries more vulnerable to injury.[88]

A research study by Brandt, et al. took skin biopsy samples from people with cervical artery dissections and reviewed them under a microscope. They found that 55% of the skin tissue samples had an underlying abnormal ultrastructural connective tissue disorder; however only 5% of those samples had a confirmed diagnosis of a known connective tissue disorder such as fibromuscular dysplasia.[89] Basically, in over half of the individuals studied with cervical artery dissections, abnormal collagen fibers in their connective tissue were present despite negative testing for known genetic tissue abnormalities.

"My neck pain started while I was exercising, and now I'm afraid to exercise because I don't want another dissection. How can I exercise safely?"

Another common theme in aggravated spontaneous dissections is overexertion during exercise. During intense exercises, your heart rate will rise in order to supply blood rich in oxygen and glucose to your muscles since your body is demanding more of these substances. It is possible that the combination of increased cardiac output combined with straining during intense exercise can result in vascular trauma.

However, keep in mind that if people stop exercising altogether, they increase the risk of obesity, high blood pressure, diabetes mellitus, and high cholesterol. These problems are much more common than dissections and can cause strokes and heart attacks. Before you begin exercising again, you should have a conversation with your healthcare provider because not all dissections are the same. In general, the majority of patients should return to a more moderate exercise regimen with time. Some patients struggle with intense fatigue after any type of exertion and have found it difficult to balance a low impact exercise regimen in their lives without triggering waves of severe pain and exhaustion. Be patient with yourself and remember that slow, gradual steps are sometimes the best way to make progress towards recovery.

"I had a healthy pregnancy, but shortly after childbirth, I had a stroke from a carotid dissection. Can labor and delivery cause a dissection?"

During a normal pregnancy, the body produces relaxin and progesterone to soften and increase the pliability of connective tissue, ligaments and joints, and is a good thing, as it will help to facilitate the delivery of the baby. Some women experience cervical artery dissection shortly after childbirth, in part, because of these changes. The excessive bearing down and straining during delivery could impact arterial structure as well. There is a need for further research to understand the association between labor and carotid and vertebral dissections.

In a literature review of 12 case studies of women who had a cervical artery dissection in the postpartum period, all 12 women presented with headache and/or neck pain.[90] The combination of increased risk for hypertension during pregnancy, hormone-induced changes of connective tissue structure, and straining during labor can all contribute to increased risk of vertebral and carotid artery dissections. A 2011 case study of a 32-year-old woman who presented with an internal carotid artery dissection, seven days after childbirth concluded that cervical artery dissection "is a condition that should be looked for in women with persisting or [unremitting] unilateral headache following childbirth."[91]

"What types of trauma can cause cervical artery dissections?"

Trauma is a common cause of carotid and vertebral dissections. Motor vehicle accidents are responsible for many cases of traumatic carotid and vertebral artery dissection. Traumatic dissections can also be caused by blunt trauma to the head and neck.

There are four types of trauma that can result in cervical artery dissection.[92] Type I dissection trauma results from a direct blow to the neck. For example, a Type I traumatic dissection could occur if a person was hit in the neck with a falling tree branch or if a patient were tackled forcibly during a football game.

Type II traumatic dissections are the most common and are a result of hyperextension and contralateral rotation of the head and neck. Examples of Type II trauma would be a car accident ("whiplash") or chiropractic cervical manipulation.

Type III traumatic dissections result from intraoral (inside the mouth) trauma. Examples of this type of dissection would be falling with a toothbrush in your mouth or experiencing a traumatic complication during oral surgery.

Type IV traumatic dissections occur with fractures in the base of the skull that include the sphenoid and petrous bones.[93] These bones line the posterior and anterior portion of the canal in which the carotid artery enters the skull.

Trauma to the vertebral arteries may result from both hyperextension and blunt trauma. The trauma mechanisms that can result in carotid dissections also apply to the vertebral arteries with the exception of intraoral penetrating traumas, which are unable to reach the vertebral arteries based on their positions. Fracture to the cervical spine (specifically the transverse process) can injure the lining of the vertebral arteries.

Where the internal carotid artery enters the skull, there is potential for injury. Damage to the skull from a car accident (closed head injury) or a bullet that penetrates the skull (open head injury) could fracture the surrounding skull and pierce the lining of the carotid artery, resulting in a dissection. Rupturing a carotid or vertebral artery is a high-risk situation for hemorrhaging and can be imminently life-threatening if not quickly addressed by a trained medical team.

Trauma to the cervical spine (levels C1 through C6) can cause damage to the linings of the vertebral arteries. The vertebral arteries travel through the transverse foramina (holes in the sides of the cervical spine), making them vulnerable to injury. The vertebral arteries are in close proximity to bony prominences of the cervical spine and the muscles and tendons that anchor them to the spine.

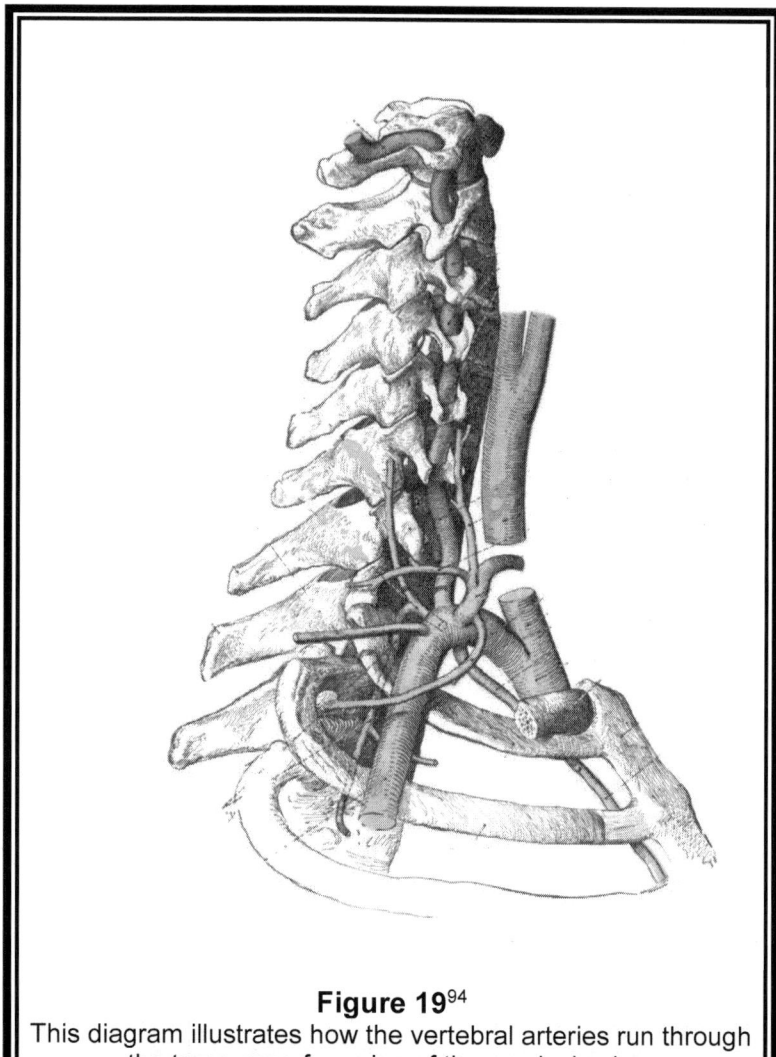

Figure 19[94]
This diagram illustrates how the vertebral arteries run through the transverse foramina of the cervical spine.

Chapter 8: Patient Story

A Couple's Perspective

Andy: Regular Font   **Melissa: Bold Font**

It was Halloween night. I stopped by the grocery store to pick up some extra candy when I got a call from Melissa saying that she was feeling weird and wanted me to come home quickly. Once I arrived, she explained that while passing out candy to some early trick-or-treaters she felt a tingling sensation in her left arm and hand and a feeling on the left side of her face like there was a hook in it pulling it back.

I remember how my left hand just started shaking uncontrollably. I even grabbed it and held it close to my body to try and make it stop. I also remember the thoughts of: "Okay, all of one side of my body, stroke, but that's old people and I'm perfectly healthy."

We debated going to the hospital but decided to see if it happened again and ate dinner. The tingling came back while we were eating, so we drove to the local emergency room. At the emergency room they spent around two hours monitoring Melissa after doing an MRI of her brain. The strange sensations never returned in the emergency room, and her vital signs were reported to us as normal.

Actually, my symptoms did return, and not saying anything is something I have regretted ever since. While lying in the bed, I saw my blanket move but couldn't figure out how. I didn't feel my hand when it moved. For some idiotic reason, maybe fear, I didn't tell anyone.

The doctor on call diagnosed it as neuropathy while stating that he'd rather be a "no man than a yes man," indicating that he didn't want to say it was something serious. Shortly after this conversation, they released Melissa.

We got home around 10:30 and went to bed around 11PM. At 11:15, I woke up and realized that something didn't feel right with Melissa. I felt her twitching in the bed. I rolled her over to face me, and that is when I saw her face. I'll never forget it - the left side of her face was drooping. I frantically woke Melissa up and said something like: "Oh my God, Melissa, your face!" I tried to get her to focus on me, but I could tell she was struggling to concentrate.

I don't remember struggling to concentrate, but I remember thinking - why was Andy making

such a fuss? I felt fine. I think I even told him I thought he was overreacting.

The entire left side of her body was paralyzed. I ran to get my phone to call 911, and while I was out of the room, Melissa tried to get up to see her face in the mirror.

Hey, I'm a girl! When someone says something about your face, you have to check it out.

When she tried to stand, she fell to the floor next to our bed. The thud was loud, and I could hear it throughout the whole house. I got back in the room and pulled her onto the bed while I spoke to 911, telling them that I thought my wife had just had a stroke. The ambulance was at our house extremely fast, but everything is a jumble of memories really. It happened very quickly, from waking up to her being loaded onto the ambulance. They rushed her back to the same emergency department, the same nurses and the same doctors. Melissa later mentioned to me that as they were rolling her through the halls to a room, she heard comments and whispers: "Is that the same girl that was in here earlier?"

Once she made it to a room where I could see her, she was awake, lucid, and was even joking around. I can't recall exactly what happened while we were in the emergency room. It was very emotional, and Melissa was very scared. I'm not sure I want to remember all of the details, to be honest. I do, however, vividly remember the doctor on the phone with the large hospital in the nearest city; I believe he was on the phone with the neurologist on call, explaining the situation and looking for direction on administering t-PA, the clot-dissolving medicine for acute stroke. We had been told about a three-hour window for t-PA, and everyone was getting increasingly anxious as time continued to pass, but nothing was being done. Finally, they decided to give Melissa the t-PA. I remember the doctor coming in with the shot and saying: "This is going to happen very fast," and it did. I watched as slowly she began to move her foot and arm, a little at a time, but you could see it was working.

Not long after the t-PA, they made the decision to transfer Melissa. Once she was there, they admitted her to the neurological ICU and began to monitor her condition. A few hours later, the neurologist gathered our family together in a room and told us what had happened. Melissa had a dissected internal carotid artery. A blood clot had formed, and eventually it broke off, causing her to have a stroke. The doctor said that the next 72 hours were going to be critical as they monitored the swelling of Melissa's brain. I asked her if Melissa could die, and she said yes, it was possible, but they weren't going to let that happen. That is when I lost it. I can only describe my reaction as hysterical. I went to an adjoining room and cried and fell to the floor, saying that I couldn't lose Melissa.

I'm talking all about myself, so Melissa will need to fill in her point-of-view. Each day got better. Melissa got better, and the swelling went away while much of her left-sided function came back to her. I think we were there for two weeks, between the Neurological ICU, a regular room, and therapy.

It's been a life-changing experience for both of us. In many ways, it made us both better people. Today Melissa still struggles with fatigue and partial paralysis of her left hand. Mentally, she battles anxiety and memory issues from the stroke.

We do get angry a lot with what-ifs. What if they hadn't sent her home? What I hadn't woken up to find Melissa? What if they had given her the t-PA sooner? I think those questions will always be around, but there isn't much we can do to answer them. They will always be there, and I hope we can eventually come to terms with them.

I was in ICU for a week. I would get confused about night and day, especially when no visitors were allowed, which I think was between 6 pm and 10 am. I hated that time. I needed someone to have eyes on me, because I was so scared of it happening again. The only reason I've been given for my dissection is that my artery may have been genetically weak, and I must have done something to tear it. I had been throwing up the week prior, so I chalk it up to that. I refuse to ever throw up again, so much so that I went an entire pregnancy without puking.

The fear of it happening again took over my life. When I got to go home, I had to have people there, not just to help me with recovery, but to be there in case it happened again. My parents would stay for a week, then my in-laws would come the next. They alternated weeks until Christmas. Once I was made to stay alone, Andy kept me up on Skype at work so I was more comfortable. I think I did that until February. I still have panic attacks for no reason from time to time.

The stroke was a blessing in disguise. It's not all sugar and honey every day. I have my moments of frustration still; it has been over five years since my stroke. It's hard on Andy having to do things that I see as stupid or trivial (pulling my hair back, tying my shoes, opening things, etc.) Sometimes I question why he would stick around, or if he's tired of it all.

BUT the good - the stroke completely changed who I am. The cynical, tomboy-ish part of me died that night, leaving a very girly, more open and loving me. I had never wanted children. I teach. I'm an elementary school librarian; I have 700 kids, why do I need another? But in my panic and anxiety and Google searches, I started to question if I could even have one. The new me began to fear that I couldn't. Did I already lose my chance at 31? My neurologist reassured me that I had not. Now, after 2 years of trying, we have a beautiful baby boy. He's truly the best thing we have ever created.

Of course, during my pregnancy, which was a rough one (four hospital stays), I worried the entire time about how was I going to take care of something so fragile with one freaking hand. Our baby, Patrick, tried coming at 29 weeks, but with rest and monitoring, he stayed until 35 weeks when he shot my blood pressure up to dangerous levels. When he arrived, those fears disappeared. I have monitored and adjusted many situations to fit our needs (hey, I am a teacher). I know I must look a fright to strangers, but he's my little boy, and I'm taking great care of him. I mean, he's alive, healthy, and always smiling. He is almost 7 months old at the time I am writing this. He is pushing 18 lbs, making it a little more of a struggle to handle him, but I'm trying my best. I tell myself I'm the only mama he knows, and he accepts me as I am. (Actually, I've had to be told that a lot to believe it myself.)

I don't feel as smart now as before, and that's bad if you're a teacher. 3rd-5th grade math shuts me down. Problems with multiple steps are especially hard for me. I can't do puzzles anymore. I have a hard time starting projects and sequencing tasks. I've been forced to be physically and mentally dependent, and I can't stand it. Being at the mercy of someone else's convenience is frustrating.

My life is definitely not easy, but it's mine. I work full time (I returned 6 months after the stroke). I have a great marriage and a beautiful child. I wouldn't trade it for anything. My only wish is for more empathy and understanding from people around me. I still have limitations and hate dealing with them. But I can't change the past.

Chapter 9:
Initial Treatment

"After my dissection, I was given a drug called Plavix. Is that enough to prevent a stroke? What is the best treatment plan?"

Diagnosing a cervical artery dissection as soon as possible is imperative to prevent stroke. Unfortunately, diagnosis and intervention for cervical artery dissection is often delayed until neurological damage is irreversible.[95] Treatment with antiplatelet therapy or anticoagulation in young patients presenting with head and neck pain stemming from cervical artery dissection can prevent stroke caused by a clot forming at the site of stenosis.[96]

Before getting into what Plavix is or when a stent may be considered, it is important to understand what a platelet is. Platelets are irregularly shaped cells in your blood that typically have a good purpose: to keep you from hemorrhaging if you were to start bleeding. Platelets "plug" the site of a wound to assist in halting bleeding when it starts. When tissue is injured, platelets come to the rescue. However, this is a problem with carotid and vertebral artery dissections, because platelets begin collecting at the dissection site, and if a platelet-rich clot becomes sizeable enough as blood is flowing around it, it can break away from the blood vessel wall and end up lodged in an artery of the brain, preventing blood flow and resulting in stroke.

Plavix (generic name: clopidogrel) helps to prevent platelets from sticking to one another and to the blood vessel wall in this scenario. Aspirin does too, but through a different mechanism. The purpose of an antiplatelet medication is to essentially prevent platelets from sticking to one another. Other oral antiplatelet medications include, but are not limited to: Aggrenox (aspirin/dipyridamole), Brilinta (ticagrelor), Pletal (cilostazol), and Effient (prasugrel). There are also IV antiplatelet therapies available too, such as Reopro (abciximab). Aspirin and/or clopidogrel are the most frequently used antiplatelet therapies to treat acute cervical artery dissection. Prasugrel should not be used if a stroke has occurred, as the FDA has labeled it with a black box warning since it was shown to place patients with stroke at high risk for bleeding in the brain. Abciximab is typically only used if stents are placed urgently to prevent platelets from adhering to the devices, but it also carries a higher risk of bleeding.

The term anticoagulant refers to medications used to prevent formation of protein-rich clots instead of targeting platelets. The best known oral anticoagulant is Coumadin (warfarin) because it has been around for decades and was largely the only oral anticoagulant available for a long time. However, the drug requires a great amount of compliance from the patient. Because the levels fluctuate in the blood, it must be monitored frequently (once a week for some patients; once a month for others), and the dose has to be adjusted if the levels are not within the desired range. It also carries higher rates of hemorrhage than aspirin, which has been demonstrated in a number of clinical trials, including WASID, a trial looking at narrowing of the arteries in the brain and stroke prevention. WASID had to be stopped early due to more frequent bleeding in patients on warfarin when compared with patients on aspirin, even though both were similarly capable of preventing strokes.[97]

There are newer oral anticoagulants that have been heavily advertised in the United States, nicknamed "NOACs" (**N**ovel **O**ral **A**nticoagulants). These include Pradaxa (dabigatran), Eliquis (apixaban), Xarelto (rivaroxaban), and Savaysa (edoxaban). These drugs have been rigorously studied in the prevention of stroke in atrial fibrillation, as well as in treating blood clots in the legs, arms, and lungs. The NOACs carry a lower risk of bleeding when compared with warfarin in patients with atrial fibrillation, but there is no meaningful data available indicating whether these drugs are effective in preventing stroke in the carotid or vertebral artery dissection population.

Heparin is an IV anticoagulant that may be used in the hospital setting by some health care providers after a dissection. It can also be injected under the skin to prevent blood clots from forming in the legs while a patient is less active than usual (lying in bed). Lovenox (generic: enoxaparin) is a form of heparin that is longer acting than unfractionated heparin (the type of heparin given through an IV), and it may be used in the outpatient setting as well.

There has been debate for many years amongst physicians who care for patients with cervical artery dissections about whether to treat patients with antiplatelet therapy or anticoagulation. The benefit of a drug like aspirin is a relatively low risk of major bleeding, but there is a question in the minds of many neurologists about whether aspirin is effective enough - "strong" enough, if you will - to prevent strokes in patients with dissections. Until recently, there was no clinical trial actually comparing antiplatelet therapy to anticoagulation in patients with carotid artery or vertebral artery dissection, and the medicine selected for treatment was based entirely on anecdotes and the bias of the treating physician.

In February of 2015, the Stroke Association of the UK published the Cervical Artery Dissection in Stroke Study (CADISS). In the CADISS trial, patients presenting to one of the participating medical centers in the United Kingdom who were diagnosed with carotid or vertebral artery dissection (with or without stroke) believed to have occurred within the seven days prior to the onset of symptoms were randomized into the study. Half of the patients were started on antiplatelet therapy, and half were placed on anticoagulation. The duration of treatment was three months. The endpoint was to determine how many strokes or deaths occurred in each group. Whether or not the patient had already had a stroke before enrolling in the trial, the endpoint was to analyze, once antiplatelet therapy or anticoagulation was started, how many patients went on to have strokes from that moment forward once they started their designated therapy.

In this study, 250 patients were enrolled (118 carotid artery dissections and 132 vertebral artery dissections). Interestingly, the investigators discovered that 52 of these patients did not actually have carotid or vertebral artery dissections when their radiological studies were carefully reviewed, despite initially receiving that diagnosis, and they were excluded.

Of the 198 patients remaining with true cervical artery dissections, there was no significant difference in strokes between the two groups. There was one episode of symptomatic bleeding in the anticoagulation group (subarachnoid hemorrhage, or bleeding in the brain that occurs when an artery in the brain ruptures). There were no deaths in either group. Of the 198 patients with radiological evidence of dissection confirmed, there were only four total strokes following initiation of the designated medical therapy in both groups combined.

The CADISS trial began as a feasibility study – a trial to see if it was even realistic to enroll enough patients with a relatively rare condition. This phase of the study was statistically sound and convincing enough not to proceed with a larger trial.

Selection of either an antiplatelet medication or an anticoagulant remains very medical provider-specific, and still stems from that provider's personal experience. Patients with these dissections will still see others with similar dissections treated with different medications. A good discussion between physician and patient of the potential risks with each therapy is very important.

The CADISS trial did not address the myriad symptoms many dissection patients notice lingering after the injury, such as migraines, neck pain, and anxiety, to name a few. One trial cannot address every possible issue associated with a medical condition. There is a strong need for ongoing research in these areas to better understand and treat dissection aftermath.

"So that is a lot of information. What are the take-away points about CADISS?"

Physicians who care for young stroke patients with this particular vascular injury should be celebrating the fact that we *finally* have evidence-based guidance for preventing stroke in these patients.

The take-away points from CADISS are as follows:

1. The great majority of patients with carotid and vertebral artery dissection, if started on either antiplatelet therapy or anticoagulation soon after the dissection has occurred, will not go on to have a stroke while on antiplatelet or anticoagulation medications during the aftermath following the vascular injury.
2. There was no significant difference in stroke prevention in patients with carotid and vertebral artery dissection between those using antiplatelet medications and those using anticoagulation.[98]

However, each patient is different. Some patients will continue to have TIAs on aspirin, and their healthcare providers have to decide whether to make a medication change. Others may have profuse bleeding on anticoagulation medications. The ultimate message of CADISS is: diagnose the dissection, and if treated with either antiplatelet therapy or anticoagulation, the patient will likely avoid stroke from that point.

"I read online in a carotid dissection support group that another patient got a stent, but this was never even mentioned to me by my neurologist when I had my carotid dissection. Should I have had a stent placed?"

A trial comparing stenting to medication alone has not been performed, and given the low number of strokes in patients on antiplatelet and anticoagulation medical therapy in the CADISS trial, it is unlikely that a dissection stenting trial will be performed any time in the near future. The CADISS study showed that medication therapy is effective the large majority of the time. Clinical trials strive to give patients the best available treatment while answering questions about management, and they should not add additional, unnecessary risk.

Put another way - the risk of stroke just from the angiogram itself (a procedure that is necessary in order to place a stent) is around 1%. In stenting trials for carotid artery disease due to plaque accumulation, the risk of stroke as a complication of a stenting procedure is as high as 3%.[99,100] The benefit from a stent would have to be so profound as to overcome the risk of the procedure, and since the risk of stroke from these dissections once treated with medical therapy is less than 3%, stents are not a mainstay of therapy. However, there are some patients who are neurologically very unstable on medical therapy, especially those who may have three or four arteries dissected, and concern may exist that these patients are still at high risk for stroke. Sometimes their physicians will decide to pursue stenting to hold the artery open and allow more optimal blood flow to the brain, even if there is a risk of stroke from the procedure. Patients who have dissected multiple arteries are a particularly difficult group to study, because this scenario is much less common than patients presenting to the hospital with a single dissection.

"When I was in the emergency department there was a great deal of discussion regarding whether or not to give me a drug called t-PA. What is it, and why don't they just automatically give it to patients experiencing signs and symptoms of a stroke?"

Tissue plasminogen activator (t-PA) occurs naturally in your body as a protein that causes blood clots to disintegrate. The drug form of t-PA (Alteplase) is a synthesized version of this and can be administered through an IV or through the tip of a catheter in an effort to dissolve a blood clot. The clinical trials evaluating IV t-PA's efficacy have been very favorable, and it is now the standard of care in patients presenting with acute ischemic stroke within the first three hours of symptom onset who are eligible to receive it. One clinical trial showed a benefit in select patients out to four and a half hours from the start of stroke symptoms.[101] In these studies, patients who received IV t-PA were more likely to be independent three months after a stroke compared with those who received placebo.[102] Decision-making around t-PA can be complicated because one of the potential adverse effects of the drug is bleeding. Therefore, patients with low platelet counts, recent bleeding, recent major surgery, or other circumstances that may result in a high risk of hemorrhaging from the drug often do not receive IV t-PA. Very high blood pressure readings may also place a patient at high risk for bleeding if t-PA is given, so if the blood pressure cannot be effectively lowered in a safe way, t-PA may be withheld. The most common reason that patients do not receive t-PA is because it cannot be given within four and a half hours of when the stroke symptoms began. If t-PA is given once a stroke has already occurred (tissue has died), the patient is unlikely to benefit from it and is at high risk for bleeding into that newly-injured area of the brain. Carotid and vertebral artery dissection patients with ischemic stroke symptoms are candidates for t-PA treatment. However, there is concern among some providers that t-PA could cause additional bleeding in the injured arterial lining, potentially causing further narrowing by increasing the size of the mural hematoma.

In reported cases in the medical literature of t-PA administered to patients with cervical artery dissection, the treatment was safe, with no subarachnoid hemorrhages or rupture of the arterial lining.[103] The American Stroke Association has also published in its guidelines that t-PA is a safe and effective form of intervention for ischemic stroke in cervical artery dissection cases, although clinical trial evidence is lacking.

"Is it possible that I could have another dissection or stroke?

After returning home from the hospital, survivors of carotid and vertebral artery dissections typically have a lot of questions and concerns. The most urgent concerns often revolve around fear of either a stroke from the current dissection or fear that another dissection will occur in the future, especially when the first dissection was spontaneous.

Studies have shown that once antiplatelet or anticoagulant therapy has been initiated, the risk of stroke after a dissection is low. The CADISS trial was discussed in detail previously. In an observational study, Steinsiepe et al reported the rate of recurrent dissection at 2 to 3.2% in the first month after the initial dissection, and then 0.3 to 1.6% per year.[104]

New dissections can occur more commonly in individuals with connective tissue disorders. It is unlikely that people with a traumatic dissection resulting from a car accident or blunt trauma will suffer another dissection since there was an inciting event that caused the vascular injury. People with spontaneous dissections from everyday activities such as overexertion from exercising or coughing may be at risk for another dissection, even though they may not have a known connective tissue disorder.

It is very unnerving to worry about having another dissection. Some neurologists recommend that patients who have had a spontaneous dissection remain on low dose aspirin if there have been no complications from the drug. In the event that another dissection does occur in the future, aspirin could reduce the risk of stroke.

"My carotid artery is blocked now because of my dissection. How long will it take to open up again?"

Survivors are frequently interested in knowing the amount of time it takes for their arteries to heal, and when completely blocked, how soon blood flow can be expected to resume. As with much of the information available regarding dissection, there is a need for further studies. Observational studies to date report that up to 90% of stenoses in cervical arteries with dissection improve to some degree.[105] Dissections with complete occlusion recanalize (open) in around 66% of cases.[106] In another smaller study, 83% of patients with anticoagulant therapy reported complete recanalization of their cervical artery occlusion after 6 months.[107]

"My doctor has me taking Coumadin (warfarin) for my vertebral artery dissection. How long should I stay on this?"

The amount of time that a patient with a carotid or vertebral artery dissection should remain on either anticoagulation or on antiplatelet therapy is not well-established and is another example of the ongoing need for more research in this area. Many neurologists will choose a select therapy for stroke prevention and continue this medication until a follow-up CT-angiogram or MR-angiogram shows at least stability of the dissection, or preferably improvement or resolution, and then will talk to the patient about stopping the therapy. Some neurologists opt to continue patients with these dissections on aspirin daily even after the vessel has "healed" on neuroimaging, in case another dissection occurs in the future. The exact period of time is not clearly specified from published data, and the practice varies between medical providers.

"My cholesterol is normal, but my primary care physician wants to put me on a statin to keep my cholesterol low. Will statins help reduce my risk of dissection, and are they necessary?"

Statins have been profoundly beneficial in preventing strokes and heart attacks by lowering cholesterol and reducing plaque accumulation. They are very effective, and a number of clinical trials have shown increased survival in patients who take them for this purpose.

The benefit of statin therapy in the carotid and vertebral artery dissection population is another unknown (and yet *another* example of the need for more research in this area). If a patient is diagnosed with a stroke, current guidelines recommend the initiation of statin therapy for stroke prevention. However, because this dissection population is typically a younger, healthier group, it is worth a discussion about whether the potential risk of statin therapy (muscular pain and cramping is the most common complaint) is justified by the possible benefit. If a patient has a dissection, but has very high LDL cholesterol, it is probably appropriate to start statin therapy to lower the LDL, and therefore lower the overall risk of stroke. If the LDL is normal or close to normal, and the stroke was caused by a traumatic dissection that arose during a car collision, then a statin may be unnecessary.

Chapter 10: Patient Story
Successful Intervention

The first notion I had that something was not right was a headache. It started out as just a headache, then it got worse. It began to pulsate around my head from back to front, and it wouldn't seem to go away for longer than an hour or two after I took Aleve. After about a week, I went into my general practitioner's office, was diagnosed with tension headaches and prescribed muscle relaxers. The very next day while I was driving to work the entire right side of my face went completely numb, and I pulled over. The feeling only lasted 45 seconds or so, and my initial thought was that it was a side effect of the muscle relaxers. I had no reason to think it was anything more serious.

For the next two days, I experienced horrible vertigo. I would get extremely dizzy and began to stumble off to the right every few hours. After this happened a few times, I decided I needed to go back to the doctor. After learning what I was experiencing, they sent me to the hospital for an MRI. As I was driving home from the MRI, my doctor called me and said the radiologists had noticed on the MRI that I had a small stroke in my cerebellum, and they needed me to drive immediately to the ER. The cerebellum controls balance and coordination, so that would explain why I was stumbling off to the right.

After quite a few tests in the ER (another MRI, an ultrasound and a CT), they were able to see where the stroke had occurred but could not determine a reason. I was transferred to a large academic hospital and admitted to the ICU for the night. At that point, I wasn't having too many effects aside from still experiencing some serious headaches. I had another MRI performed around midnight that night, and at 3:00 AM. I was awakened by hospital staff and told I needed to be rushed into emergency surgery. On the last MRI, they saw that I had bilateral vertebral artery dissections and both arteries were completely occluded.

The surgery performed was a balloon angioplasty, and it went as well as could be hoped. I was very lucky! Coming out of the procedure I was placed on a heparin drip and was in the ICU for about 5 days. The main effects I had during that time were a severe headache, difficulty swallowing, weakness in my limbs, and I was unable to feel pain or temperature on my right side. I required a tube in my nose to push medication and food until my swallowing improved, and my strength slowly returned as well.

The only lasting side effect I have had is the lack of sensation of pain and temperature in my right side, including my right arm and my right leg. As I write this, it has been about five months now since my stroke and those sensations have not yet returned. Other than that I feel I have made a full recovery. I have been on Plavix and low-dose aspirin since leaving the hospital, and I took Lyrica until the headaches wore off (for about a month total).

I was out of work for about three weeks following my return home, but since then have resumed my job and daily exercise, as well as most activities I enjoyed leading up to my stroke and the procedure. I consider myself very lucky and am thankful I was in the hands of great doctors and nurses. I am also glad that I decided to go to the doctor in the first place, as it is something I normally tend to push off as long as possible!

Chapter 11:
Pain

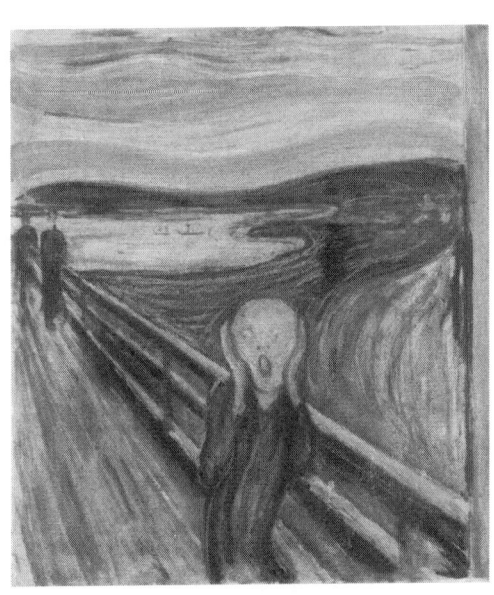

Figure 20[108]

The Scream by Edvard Munch may represent how some carotid and vertebral artery dissection patients feel when they are experiencing pain.

"Can an injury to a carotid or vertebral artery be painful?"

Yes! The walls of the carotid arteries are closely intertwined with a complex network of autonomic nerves, known as the sympathetic chain.

The cervical arteries are innervated with nerve fibers that sense pain when triggered. These nerve fibers can result in severe headaches if the artery sustains damage.[109]

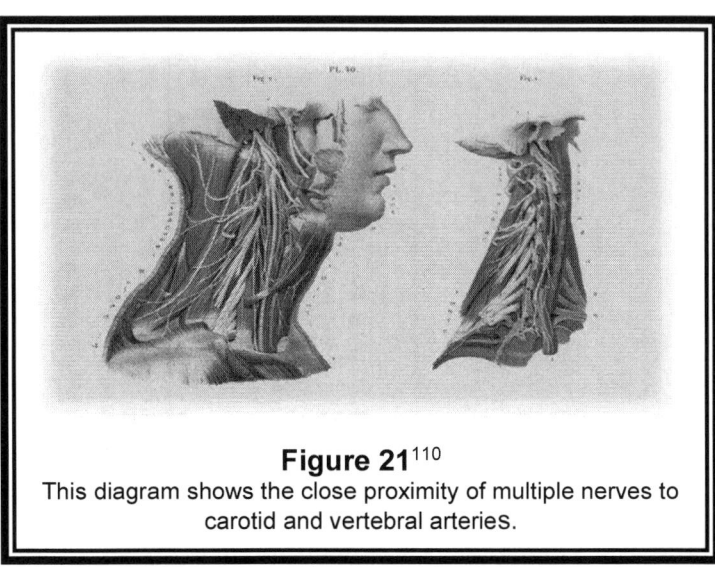

Figure 21[110]
This diagram shows the close proximity of multiple nerves to carotid and vertebral arteries.

It is beneficial for survivors of cervical artery dissection, as well as the medical professionals who provide their care, to understand that dissections can result in long-term head and neck pain. Chronic pain in dissection patients is not often recognized, which can lead to frustration on the part of patients. More research is needed to better know how to effectively treat this pain.

"Why am I having chronic head and neck pain even though my artery has "healed"?

Follow-up CT-angiography or MR-angiography may reveal that a previously dissected carotid or vertebral artery has "healed," meaning that blood flow is no longer being blocked or narrowing may no longer be present. "Healed" does not mean "normal" or "as it was before." Consider a severe skin wound that has healed and left a scar. Like the skin, a "healed" artery and the area affected will not be the same as it was before the dissection. The unfortunate truth is that pain can linger in patients with these dissections for many years following the vascular injury, which can create a sense of hopelessness in patients as they suffer. Participating in support groups and finding an empathetic and attentive pain specialist to help with symptoms are both critical.

It has been well-established that pain is one of the most prominent symptoms of acute vertebral and carotid artery dissection. When the lining of the cervical arteries endure trauma, the artery can sense pain and severe head and neck pain result. Both the vertebral and carotid arteries have a complex layer of nerves intertwined within the arteries.

There is a lack of research regarding why cervical artery dissections result in cases of severe

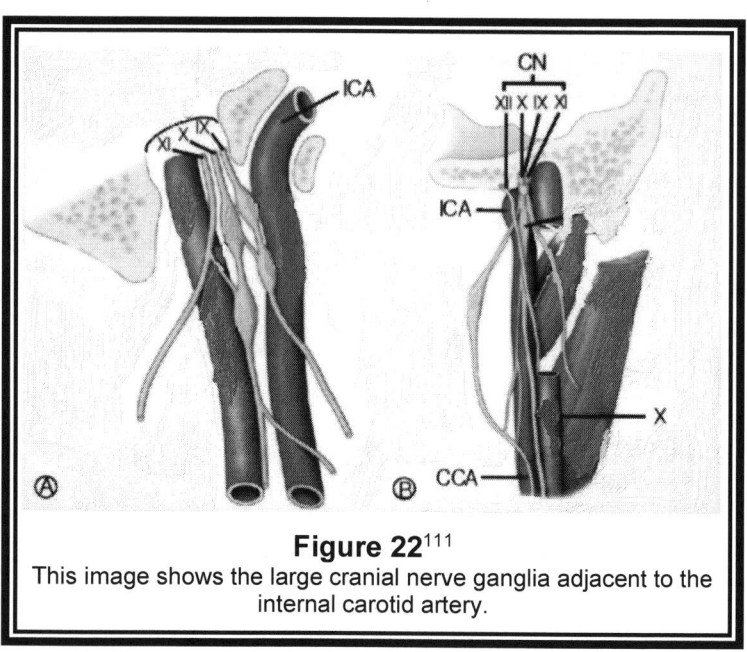

Figure 22[111]
This image shows the large cranial nerve ganglia adjacent to the internal carotid artery.

chronic pain. The adjacent sympathetic plexus of nerves, the cranial nerves, and impacted intracranial vasculature may all contribute to a variety of symptoms of pain and hypersensitivity. [112]

There are no research studies that have analyzed survivors of carotid and vertebral dissections with chronic pain. Until adequate research is completed, there will be little to no knowledge of what to tell patients to expect and which treatments might be the most effective.

Another rationale for chronic pain after a dissection is that when the artery dissects, the location of nerves and the artery shift, resulting in tissue that could come into more direct contact with the surrounding nerves. While most cases of trigeminal neuralgia do not arise from vascular dissections, it is an example of an extremely painful condition that can come about from physical contact of an artery or other structure with the trigeminal nerve, resulting in either constant or severe episodes of facial pain. Contact between structures and the trigeminal nerve can compress the nerve and wear away at the protective coating (myelin sheath) around the nerve.[113] The American Association of Neurological Surgeons notes that trigeminal neuralgia is sometimes described as "the most excruciating pain known to humanity."[114] This type of severely painful compression of nerves can be a possible result of cervical dissections.

Another theory for why chronic pain after a cervical artery dissection exists involves a change in the artery's ability to appropriately constrict and relax. Neurons in the brain do not sense pain, but the thin tissue covering on the brain (the meninges) can sense pain.

Sometimes the pain that patients experience following cervical artery dissections is migraine. Migraine is a vascular syndrome in which blood flow patterns shift, activation of the trigeminal nucleus in the brainstem can occur, and severe headaches can result. Migraine can be extremely disabling for cervical artery dissection patients.

Some people who have had a dissection and suffer from chronic pain could be experiencing pain memory. In some cases, the nerves continue to sense pain even though the original trigger is no longer present.[115] The nerves can be stuck in a continuous cycle of triggering pain, which can result in hypersensitivity to pain.

Cervical dissections can also cause musculoskeletal pain. After an injury, it is the body's natural response for muscles to tighten around the damaged area. Patients with cervical artery dissections may be overly cautious about moving their necks, and over time, this spasticity can result in a reduction in the neck's range of motion with an increase in muscular tension.

"What should I do if my doctor doesn't believe I am in pain?"

(From: *The Stroke Blog*, November 15, 2014)

Pain is a subjective experience, and it differs from person to person. My sympathy for the carotid and vertebral dissection patient populations is great because the pain can be so unrelenting. However, because many of these patients look so normal externally, they are sometimes not believed when they describe the severity of their pain.

My pain during routine dental visits and procedures is unreal at times, and I have stopped trying to explain to others how much suffering I endure in that situation because no one around me really believes it. Perhaps I am just not tough enough. Perhaps my "pain threshold" is low. Whatever. The pain, as I experience it, is real, and it is awful. However, my dentist is a kind, empathetic person who believes me, and a little empathy goes a long way.

I know that patients who experience pain on a daily basis that nears or exceeds the severity of the pain I endure in the dental office might feel a little more hopeful if the physician who is supposed to be treating them believes that their pain is real.

The relationship between a healthcare provider and a patient is based on trust, and so it is important to find someone to provide your care in whom you can place yours. Ask friends and family for recommendations. Online support groups can be a good source for seeking recommendations, too.

"Since my dissection was on the left side, why was my headache on both sides of my head?"

There are several reasons why this could be the case. The dissection could have triggered a migraine with more diffuse headache pain. The neck stiffness in response to the dissection could have also resulted in a more generalized tension headache.

It is also crucial to remember that cervical artery dissections can occur on both sides. Patients may present to the emergency department or to their primary care providers with both carotid arteries and/or both vertebral arteries dissected.

Overall, the pain is generally on the same side as the dissection if only one dissection is present.[116] However, it is not uncommon for patients with one cervical artery dissection to experience diffuse headaches.

"What are some preventative pain medications I should ask my doctor about?"

First of all, there are two different core strategies for treating pain with medications: preventative medications and abortive pain medications. The goal of preventative medicine is to decrease the frequency of painful episodes and the intensity of the pain when a painful episode starts. Abortive pain medications combat pain once it has begun. For patients who have painful episodes infrequently, it may make more sense for them just to have medicine to use abortively once pain starts, rather than risk side effects from a daily preventative medication that may not provide as much benefit.

If a patient experiences consistent pain and has to use abortive pain medications with regularity, then a regular preventative medication may be a reasonable option. In selecting the right medication, it is important to define what the source of the pain is. For example, if a patient with a vertebral artery dissection is experiencing severe muscular spasms in the neck and shoulders, it may not make sense to use a migraine preventative medication.

"My doctor started me on a medicine called amitriptyline (Elavil) for my migraines after my dissection. It's an antidepressant, but I don't feel depressed. Why would she give me an antidepressant if I am not depressed?"

Amitriptyline (Elavil) is a tricyclic antidepressant medication that has been around for decades. Currently, it is prescribed for the management of chronic pain, including pain associated with headaches and neuropathy (nerve pain in the feet and/or hands). It also can be used to help with sleep disturbances. It is not uncommon that patients with headaches are also not sleeping adequately, and many healthcare providers will use this medication to try to alleviate both problems. It is often recommended that amitriptyline be taken at night.

A number of clinical studies have evaluated the effectiveness of amitriptyline in treating migraines, and the findings are favorable. In a retrospective study, 75% of patients (134 out of 178) reported some improvement in headaches after starting the medication, and 85% of patients were still taking it at their most recent follow-up appointment.[117] The high level of compliance speaks to the medication generally being well-tolerated in terms of side effects. However, no medication is perfect, and amitriptyline does have potential side effects. The most common include fatigue, drowsiness (in particular feeling sleepy in the mornings after the first days of adjusting to it), dry mouth, constipation, and the potential for worsening depression symptoms. Please talk to your healthcare provider about specifics pertaining to your care if you have concerns about a possible side effect.

To answer the question asked, though, amitriptyline is prescribed very frequently to patients for headache management who have no history of depression, and who are not currently depressed.

"I recently started topiramate (Topamax) for my migraines, but I am afraid to stay on it because I have been reading about the side effects."

Topiramate (Topamax) is an anticonvulsant medication which is used to control seizures, but can also be very effective in preventing migraine attacks. Just like any medication, though, topiramate can result in side effects. Patients complain that they cannot focus as intently, or that their concentration and short-term memory seem impaired. Individuals may feel "foggy" mentally on topiramate, but others may not experience this symptom. Another common side effect is a tingling sensation in fingers and toes. Often this feeling stops as a person's body adjusts to the medication, but sometimes the tingling sensation persists, and patients decide to stop taking topiramate because the negative side effects outweigh the benefits.

Patients with a history of recurrent kidney stones or glaucoma probably should not take this medication, as topiramate can worsen these conditions. A discussion with your healthcare provider is especially important.

There are other side effects associated with topiramate as well, which are available in the medicine's package insert and online, but those mentioned here are the more common ones. If you have concerns, please speak openly with your healthcare provider about them.

This being said, many patients who have been suffering with refractory migraines for years have found great relief on topiramate. The benefit provided by any drug must be balanced with the potential for harm (side effects), and if the balance falls in favor of the benefit provided, then sometimes it is worth using. Every individual is unique in his or her response to a medication, though, and specifics of a situation should be considered in each case.

"My neurologist recommended gabapentin for my headaches and neck pain and wants me to eventually get up to 600 mg three times a day. That sounds like a lot! Is it?"

Believe it or not, it may not be. Some patients feel fatigued or sedated on even 100mg of gabapentin three times daily, and others use 1200mg three times daily with good pain relief and no sedation. Gabapentin is another medication that was developed to prevent
seizures, but it can also be very effective at helping to alleviate chronic pain.

Among the anti-seizure medications, the American Academy of Neurology classifies topiramate and divalproex sodium (Depakote) as top level recommendations for migraine prevention, based on the amount of scientific evidence demonstrating efficacy.

There is less evidence supporting the use of gabapentin, and side effects have to be considered. For example, divalproex sodium is known to potentially result in bone density loss in some people, so it may not always be a good option for postmenopausal women. A patient may feel too cognitively impaired on topiramate, and gabapentin may be a reasonable next choice.

"I've heard mixed things about using the medication Imitrex for migraine pain after a dissection. Is it safe?"

Sumatriptan (the trade name is Imitrex) is a migraine abortive medication that is available as a nasal spray, an oral tablet, or an injection. Sumatriptan is not intended to prevent migraines, but is used as an abortive pain medication after the onset of migraine.

To put it simply, during a migraine, blood flow increases to the brain. Sumatriptan works by causing blood vessels throughout the brain to constrict, holding back some of that extra blood flow. If you have a blocked artery from a dissection, or an artery that is already narrow and blood is struggling to get through that tight area, sumatriptan would generally not be recommended

Another risk associated with taking triptans for migraine relief is the potential interaction with some antidepressant medications. The FDA issued a public health advisory warning of the interaction of triptans with certain antidepressants, both SSRIs (selective serotonin reuptake inhibitors), and SNRIs (serotonin-norepinephrine reuptake inhibitors).

Taking sumatriptan while on antidepressants can lead to serotonin syndrome, a set of symptoms and changes that occur in the body when serotonin levels are too high. These include, but are not limited to, rapid heartbeat, sudden changes in blood pressure, increased body temperature, restlessness, overactive reflexes, hallucinations, loss of coordination, nausea, vomiting, and diarrhea. Serotonin syndrome is a medical emergency that requires immediate medical attention.[118] Antidepressants that may have this interaction with triptans include citalopram (Celexa), duloxetine (Cymbalta), escitalopram (Lexapro), fluoxetine (Prozac, Sarafem), fluvoxamine (Luvox), paroxetine (Paxil), sertraline (Zoloft), and venlafaxine (Effexor), but this list is not fully comprehensive. Serotonin syndrome is extremely dangerous and further illustrates the need for comprehensive discussions with your medical provider and careful follow-up with your pharmacist.

"Are there any procedures that can help relieve my head and neck pain that don't involve taking medicine every day?"

There are multiple nerve blocks and injections that can help relieve head and neck pain.

A trigger point is an area within the muscles that causes pain when pressure is applied that travels to another location. A trigger point can produce headaches as well. At times, trigger point tenderness can result in severe pain, and it can be challenging to achieve relief with oral medications. Trigger point injections involve injecting local anesthetic medication sometimes in combination with a corticosteroid at the site of tenderness. In one study, 86% of providers reported patients getting relief from neck pain and headache symptoms with trigger point injections.[119] The duration of relief varies between patients. Some report only very short-term relief (hours to days), while others may have months during which they are pain-free. The benefits of trigger point injections include safety, fewer daily side effects, and, if effective, avoiding dependence on substances such as narcotics.

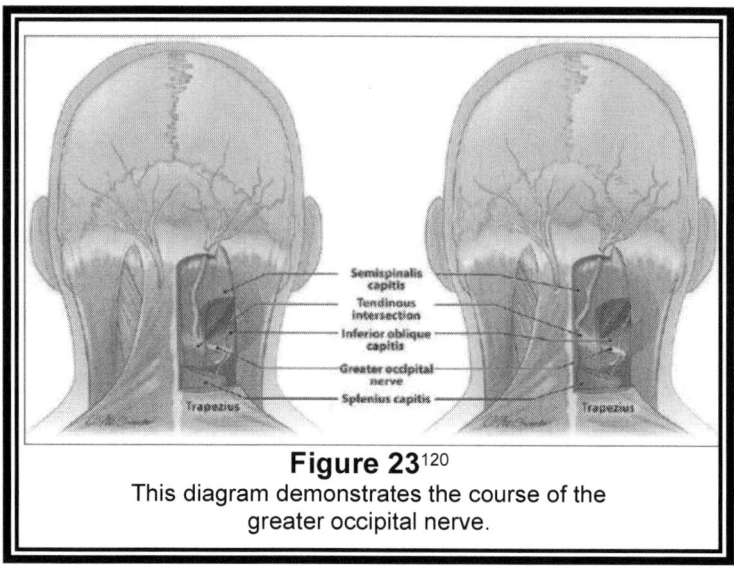

Figure 23[120]
This diagram demonstrates the course of the greater occipital nerve.

Greater occipital nerve (GON) blocks are a series of injections for pain relief. There are two greater occipital nerves (one on each side) that run from the back of the head up to the forehead and register sensation, including pain for most of the back and top of the head. GON blocks temporarily provide anesthetic medication via injection along the paths of the greater occipital nerves. Excitability of the greater occipital nerves can result in pain from the base of the skull up to the top of the head and temples. GON blocks can alleviate this excitability, leading to a reduction in muscular tension for temporary pain relief. Again, some patients will experience relief for months, while others may see benefit for shorter periods of time or not at all.

Sufferers of chronic head and neck pain can experience excessive muscle tension. Individuals with vertebral artery dissections tend to have more localized pain at the backs of their heads and necks and may benefit from GON blocks. Other more permanent techniques also exist, such as surgically decompressing the nerve or deliberately causing permanent damage to the greater occipital nerves using a toxin or radio-frequency.[121]

Acupuncture is a therapy based in traditional Chinese medicine that places thin needles in specific locations in the skin to help reduce frequency, duration, and intensity of headaches and migraines. These acupoints are believed to have a higher concentration of nerves. Some neurologists administer acupuncture for chronic neurological pain. The available reviews of clinical studies that examine the efficacy of acupuncture treatment for chronic migraine and headache have concluded that acupuncture can be a helpful form of pain reduction.[122] Additional studies are needed to examine long-term relief and impact on a wider range of head and neck pain.[123]

Acupressure is similar to acupuncture but without the use of needles. The idea is to apply pressure manually to specific points throughout the body to release endorphins and to assist in promoting pain relief.[124] Acupressure can improve blood flow, relax muscles, and reduce stress. As long as pressure to acupoints does not cause discomfort and avoids areas directly above cervical arteries, there are limited precautions with these therapies.

Acupressure has been successful in clinical trials in reducing headaches, and in a small but promising study, acupressure was found to be more effective than muscle relaxant medication to reduce the negative impact of chronic headaches on quality of life.[125]

"Is it safe to see a physical therapist for neck pain?"

Physical therapists can help with weakness resulting from stroke as well as treat chronic pain. Physical therapy utilizes a wide variety of modalities to help improve range of motion, reduce muscle tension, improve strength and reduce pain.

Physical therapy can be an excellent way to address neck pain, especially if you have muscle tension and difficulty turning your head from side to side.

"I have been avoiding massage therapy since my vertebral artery dissection out of concern that I could end up with another dissection. Is massage therapy okay?"

Massage therapy is generally considered safe for patients who have sustained carotid or vertebral artery dissections. As is the case with any therapy, caution is advised with the amount of pressure applied over the carotid arteries during the massage. The vertebral arteries are not actively palpated during massage therapy because they are surrounded by bone. Cervical manipulative therapy should be avoided in patients who have had cervical arterial dissections. Please refer back to page 119 for more information.

Cranial sacral therapy is a type of massage that addresses the bones of the head and spine. At first glance, this may seem like it would be off limits for dissection survivors, but it is actually an extremely gentle therapy. The massage is designed to hardly touch the skin and apply less pressure than that of laying a small coin over the area of focus. When performed correctly, cranial sacral therapy can be relaxing and can provide some stress and pain relief.

The therapies and injections mentioned are meant to provide supplemental relief and should never substitute for medical care or replace your medication for prevention of stroke.

"I noticed swimmers in the Olympics using cupping therapy to help with tight muscles. Is this safe to use for my dissection pain?"

No! There have been several documented cases of cupping therapy actually causing cervical artery dissections.[126,127] Cupping therapy creates suction and causes your blood vessels to expand. If placed above an artery, the force from the suction can lead to a separation of arterial walls, potentially resulting in a dissection and possibly stroke. Cupping is not a safe option for dissection survivors.

"I heard that Botox can be used to prevent headache pain. I thought it was just for wrinkles. How does it work to reduce pain?"

Another option for chronic pain after carotid and vertebral dissection is botulinum toxin. Botox is a botulinum toxin product with wide name recognition, but other products containing botulinum toxin exist as well. Botulinum toxin is an FDA-approved prescription medication administered in injection form. It is indicated for individuals who have migraines that last longer than 4 hours for at least 15 days each month. The insurance approval process can be quite lengthy. Typically, insurance companies will require proof that you have tried other medications to help alleviate your pain before coverage is approved for botulinum toxin.

Acetylcholine is a chemical released from the ends of nerves needed to trigger the contraction of muscle fibers. Botulinum toxin binds to the nerve and reduces the release of acetylcholine, paralyzing muscle fibers since they are unable to contract. The injections begin to work for most patients within four to six days, and therapeutic effects typically last for about three months.[128]

Depending on the location and quantity of injections, you may have limited facial muscle movements. Some patients are unable to move their eyebrows or furrow their eyebrows after these injections. Some individuals with chronic pain resulting from cervical artery dissection find that botulinum injections reduce the severity of their headaches and muscle tension, but typically it is not a "cure." It is one of many approaches used to help make life manageable with chronic pain.

"I've tried over a dozen different preventative pain medications, and nothing helps. I can't function because of the pain. The only time I get any relief is when I take an opioid. Is this a viable option for long term pain relief?"

If your pain has impacted your quality of life and stopped you from being able to work and participate in desired activities, opiate pain medication may be an option. It is imperative that you try multiple types of preventative pain medication before you resort to using narcotics.

Common opiate pain medications include:
- Codeine
- Hydrocodone
- Oxycodone
- Fentanyl
- Hydromorphone
- Meperidine
- Methadone
- Morphine

Opiates are highly addictive and over time become less effective at lower doses as tolerance develops. If you have a personal history of addiction or a family history of addiction, it may be in your best interest to avoid opiates completely. On the other hand, pain from cervical artery dissections can be unbearable, and if opiates are the only form of relief that works for you, the benefits of being able to participate in activities with a break from pain may outweigh the risks. This issue is worth a thoughtful and honest discussion with your healthcare provider.

There is no set timeline for when cervical artery dissections will stop causing pain. Some members of dissection support groups have been battling pain for over a decade. It is unlikely that opiate pain medication will be able to effectively relieve your pain indefinitely. Your body will build up a tolerance and will need more medication to provide relief. Also, even without abuse, opiates will lead to physical dependence, so at some point when the medication becomes less effective, it may be difficult (even painful) to wean yourself off of narcotics.

Long-term use of opiate medication will also deplete your body of the ability to produce your own endorphins to combat pain. Research shows that long-term opiate use can lead to hyperalgesia (an increased sensitivity to pain). Although narcotic pain management may help initially, eventually it can actually increase your pain levels and deplete your body of its ability to provide natural pain relief, making chronic pain even worse.

If you do start long-term opiates, keep a journal of your pain levels. Be aware of when your pain medication becomes less effective at reducing your pain and how often you have to increase the dose for the same results. Clinical studies have shown that patients on high levels of opiates actually experienced a reduction in pain when they reduced their opiate intake.[129]

Typically, narcotic pain medication should not be prescribed for chronic headaches or migraines, but dissection survivors know that dissection pain can be extremely debilitating and refractory. When considering long-term opiate pain medication, you might want to discuss your options with several different providers. Make sure you feel comfortable with your healthcare provider, because switching between providers for narcotic medications can be difficult.[130]

If you have tried many different preventative pain medications and procedures with little success, narcotic pain management may be an option for you. Weigh the potential risks and benefits of these medications.

"Ever since my dissection, bright lights are painful to be around and give me headaches. Is this normal?"

Photophobia (sensitivity to light) is a common symptom after cervical artery dissection and also a classic feature of many migraine presentations. One patient with a left internal carotid artery dissection said, "Bright lights that shine in my left eye cause a stabbing pain like an ice pick in my eye and the pain level is about an 8 out of 10 and can last for 3 hours. Fluorescent lights make me feel like a weight is crushing the left side of my head, and the longer I am under the lights, the more severe it becomes. It takes about an hour of rest in dim lighting for the pain to dissipate."

Phonophobia (sensitivity to sound) is another common migraine symptom that can arise after these dissections.

Keeping the lights and noise level low in your home can help improve your comfort level. If you wear glasses, you can get specially tinted glasses to block excessive light. Also, effective treatment of underlying migraines that are causing the photophobia and phonophobia may effectively diminish or resolve these symptoms.

"I have started to avoid going to restaurants, parties and big gatherings because I can't handle the noise. Is there anything that can help me?"

Cervical artery dissection survivors often experience hypersensitivity to noise. Noise from parties, restaurants, children, and crowds can be very difficult to tolerate. Sound reduction earplugs can help decrease painful background noise.

An audiologist can custom fit the earplugs to your ears by making a wax mold of your ear canal. The earplugs reduce background noise but still allow you to have a conversation. Unfortunately, these are not typically covered by health insurance plans.

Soft, pliable, over-the-counter earplugs can also be effective. They are inexpensive and are usually quite comfortable.

"What else can I try to help reduce my pain?"

Cervical artery dissection survivors tend to get creative in ways to help relieve their pain since it can be so relentless. You may want to give some home remedies a try, especially if you are having trouble finding an effective medication regimen.

Heating pads and ice packs can be a helpful way to combat headaches. Adequate hydration is especially important for cervical artery dissections where narrowing in the artery still exists. Dehydration can trigger migraines and headaches as well as cause dizziness, weakness, and fainting.

Peppermint extract can be soothing. You can mix a few drops of peppermint oil with olive oil or water and rub the solution on your forehead. Be careful not to put undiluted peppermint extract directly on your skin. You can also use fresh crushed peppermint leaves instead of extract. Mint chapstick can also feel good on your skin, and it is already diluted. You can add peppermint oil to the outside of your ice or heat pack, as well. Peppermint also can be soothing as a steam treatment. Add a few drops of peppermint oil to boiling water and enjoy the aroma.

Lavender has been recognized for its soothing effects and ability to promote sleep. It also can be used to help relieve headache pain. In one clinical study, 92 out of 129 people who inhaled lavender for 15 minutes after the onset of a headache experienced at least partial pain relief.[131]

Interestingly, a clinical study compared ginger to sumatriptan, a migraine abortive medication discussed previously on page 177. Improvement in pain was demonstrated with both ginger and sumatriptan.[132]

Basil can serve as a muscle relaxant. Research has shown that basil and clove oil can relax smooth muscle tissue.[133] Cloves can also be used to relieve tension headaches. You can crush fresh cloves, keep them in a handkerchief, and smell the cloth when headache pain is present. Clove oil mixed with olive oil or coconut oil can also be rubbed on your temples and forehead to help relieve pain.

Many cervical artery dissection survivors find rest essential to help manage their pain. After a brain injury, patients often feel fatigued, and it is essential to give yourself time to recharge. When you are in pain, try to create a quiet environment. A dark cool room can help reduce the intensity of pain.

Using alternative medicine isn't a cure-all and may only be minimally helpful, but anything that helps reduce pain and tension and promotes relaxation safely should be considered.

Chapter 12: Patient Story

Exhausted

On a Sunday night in October of 2014, I was getting ready for the work week. I heard the dryer start, and I asked my husband: "Who is using the dryer?"

He said, "No one. It's not even on."

An hour or so later, I asked him the same thing. He said again that the dryer was off. Turns out it was the pulse in my ear I was hearing.

I kind of blew it off, until the end of the week when the pulsatile sound was so loud, even my husband could hear it.

I initially went to urgent care. The doctor said it was probably the start of an ear infection and if it got worse, to come back. Since I wasn't able to get into my regular doctor after another week, I went back to urgent care. The pulse in my ear was so loud, I couldn't hear what people were saying. The urgent care doctor told me to go to an ENT doctor. So, I did. He said he had no idea what it was, that maybe it was an ear infection.

Then I had a migraine headache that wouldn't go away. I was in bed with tons of ice on my head. I called my husband, and he took me to ER. The ER doctor listened to my symptoms and sent me for a CT scan of my head. The CT was normal, so he gave me a prescription for antibiotics for a possible ear infection.

I was finally able to see my regular physician. She listened to my symptoms. She said, "Something's not right." She ordered an MRI that day. When the results returned, a neurologist contacted me and asked me to come in.

I was diagnosed with a carotid artery dissection on my right side. I was told to take aspirin, and I would be rechecked in 6 months.

On my six month follow up MRI, I was told that there has been no change except that there was a pseudoaneurysm as well then. At my one year MRI, I was told the same thing.

The symptoms I have experienced (some on a daily basis) are headaches, migraines, pulsatile tinnitus, memory issues. The biggest is fatigue. I never took time off of work. I have been a middle school health/physical education teacher for 29 years.

I went to my regular doctor and left feeling as though my concerns about fatigue, memory issues, headaches were not taken seriously.

I went to see my neurologist to see if he would take my symptoms seriously. I had everything written down: the extreme fatigue, memory issues, pulsatile tinnitus, and migraines. Long story short, when I explained my symptoms, and how many of the people from my online dissection support group had the same symptoms, he said that those symptoms weren't from a dissection.

He kept asking me about my diet, my sleep, my caffeine intake, and my exercise habits. I told him: "I'm a PE and health teacher. I have my Masters in Health Science. I don't drink, I don't smoke, I don't drink coffee. I try to exercise, but I'm so exhausted at the end of the work day that's it's really tough."

He told me that my symptoms were probably from not getting a full night's sleep and that I was probably depressed. He went on to say that I was probably in denial, but that there was nothing to be ashamed of.

I told him that I teach this stuff, and I know what depression is. I'm not depressed. I'm exhausted. Then I told him, as tears ran down my face, that I was leaving because if I didn't, I may say things that I might regret later.

It's so frustrating. I'm not making up my symptoms, and when I feel like my doctor and my neurologist don't believe me, I just don't know what else to do. I hope to find a doctor/neurologist that truly understands carotid dissections and the symptoms that can follow them.

Chapter 13:
Aftermath Symptoms
Anxiety, Depression, Fatigue, and Cognitive Changes

"I never had problems with anxiety before my carotid artery dissection, but now I feel anxious constantly. What has happened?"

It is not uncommon for people who have sustained carotid and vertebral artery dissections to experience symptoms of anxiety, even if it has not existed previously. These patients may also have panic attacks for the first time in their lives. Anxiety can result as a natural emotional response to the trauma of the cervical artery dissection. After all, this vascular injury is nowhere on a young, healthy person's radar, and suddenly a whole new level of vulnerability enters the picture. That alone is enough reason to feel anxious. Often cervical artery dissection patients, especially soon after the injury, feel anxious about whether another dissection will occur.

Direct physical damage to the sympathetic nervous system can also occur with a carotid artery dissection. The sympathetic nervous system regulates our fight-or-flight responses and when triggered by trauma can create surges of hormones released during times of extreme stress.

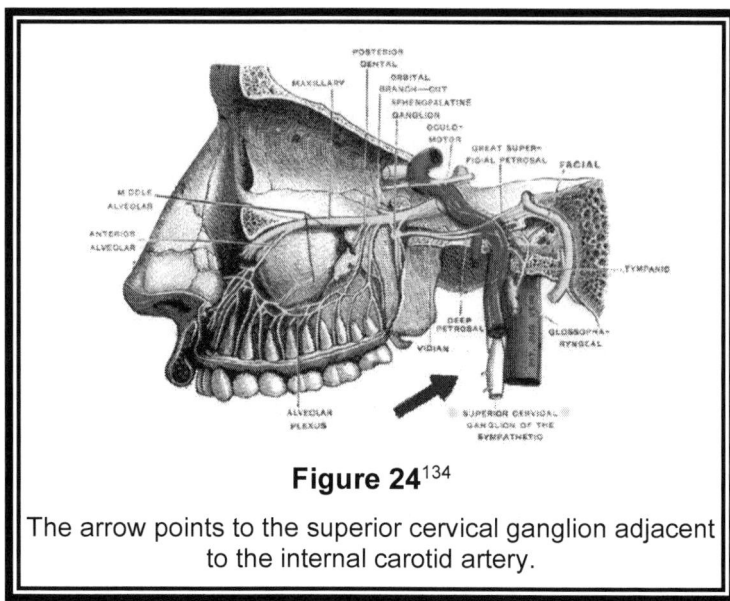

Figure 24[134]
The arrow points to the superior cervical ganglion adjacent to the internal carotid artery.

When you look at Figure 24, notice the close proximity of the superior cervical ganglion of the sympathetic nervous system and the internal carotid artery.

Anxiety is common following a stroke, especially in the younger stroke population. Younger patients are not expecting a stroke to derail their lives, and this event can prove very distressing. Additionally, after a brain injury, surges of stress hormones (cortisol, epinephrine, norepinephrine) may occur, which can result in panic attacks in patients with no prior psychiatric history.

Anxiety should probably be managed early so that it does not escalate. If your anxiety is severe enough and a primary care provider or a neurologist does not feel comfortable managing it, then assistance from psychiatry should be sought. Patients may feel they will be labeled in a negative way by seeking care from a psychiatrist, but this is a stigma that needs to end. Counseling may also be recommended. Not only can carotid and vertebral dissections be emotionally traumatic, but brain injuries can result in hormone and chemical disturbances that can cause profound mood symptoms.

"Ever since my carotid dissection, sometimes my heart starts pounding, and I have a surge of overwhelming anxiety and I feel like I can't breathe. I'm terrified. What is happening to me?"

A panic attack is an episode of intense fear, anxiety, and discomfort that can include very unpleasant symptoms, including palpitations, accelerated heart rate, sweating, shaking, shortness of breath, choking, chest pain, nausea, dizziness, lightheadedness, chills, numbness, tingling, the sensation of being separated from oneself (dissociation), and intense fear of losing control.

A panic attack can be terrifying and make you feel as if you are having a heart attack or even dying. While exercise can sometimes help to reduce the severity and frequency of panic attacks, unfortunately, panic attacks are not events you can necessarily will yourself to ignore, and often patients need proper medical therapy to manage these episodes. If you continue to experience panic attacks, you should talk with your healthcare provider about adjusting your medication regimen. When you experience one, try to remember that your sympathetic nervous system is setting off a false alarm (remember that "fight-or-flight" response), making you feel as if you are in danger. Try taking deep breaths and let a family member know what is happening to you.

"My dissection has turned my life upside down. I suffer from anxiety and depression. Can this be post-traumatic stress disorder?"

Stroke and cervical artery dissection survivors can suffer from post-traumatic stress disorder (PTSD). There are degrees of trauma, and cervical artery dissection is indeed traumatic, both physically and emotionally. PTSD symptoms include nightmares, flashbacks to the event, avoidance of places and events that remind the individual of the trauma, feelings of guilt and shame, insomnia, intense fear with elevated heart rate, and high blood pressure.[135]

One of the hallmark symptoms of PTSD is the inability to continue with daily activities because of immobilization from fear and anxiety.[136] PTSD can be isolating and remove an individual from enjoying social situations.

Approximately one in four people who survive a TIA or a stroke suffer from PTSD.[137] There have only been a few studies examining the prevalence of PTSD in TIA and stroke patients, and some of them exclude individuals with aphasia and cognitive deficits, so PTSD may actually more common than reported.[138] Studies have also found that PTSD can occur after a TIA, not just a stroke.[139] Many cervical artery dissection patients have experienced TIAs and/or strokes as part of their presentations.

The National Stroke Association recognizes that one in four stroke survivors suffer from PTSD. Having a support network of mental health professionals, family members, and friends is a valuable way to help with symptoms of PTSD. Support groups can be especially therapeutic.

In a study that specifically looked at survivors of cervical artery dissection and factors associated with PTSD, 45% of the study's participants with cervical artery dissections met the diagnostic criteria for PTSD compared to about 2% of the general population.[140]

"I keep having fainting spells, especially if I overexert myself. Is this related to my dissection?"

The carotid arteries are actually very fascinating vessels. They contain structures called carotid bodies (one on each side) just beyond the point at which the common carotid artery splits into the internal and external carotid arteries. The carotid bodies are filled with receptors that detect changes in oxygen and carbon dioxide content in the blood, and feed this information back to the medulla (the lower portion of the brainstem). The medulla then helps to regulate blood pressure, heart rate, and respiratory rate to help maintain consistent levels of these gases.

If there is an injury to the carotid body on the side of the carotid artery dissection, it is feasible that fainting spells could occur if blood pressure is poorly regulated. Often when we are sitting or lying down, when we change positions to stand abruptly there can be a delay of several seconds to keep blood flow to the brain consistent. If the carotid body is damaged, this may be more problematic.

Additionally, if an artery is blocked or if severe narrowing is present because of a dissection, and the brain is dependent on collateral flow (flow from other sources), pressure is needed to distribute this additional blood flow. If this mechanism for regulating blood pressure is impaired, this can result in fainting.

"After my dissection, I feel exhausted all the time. Every little activity tires me out. My grandparents have more energy than I do. Why am I so tired?"

Many survivors of cervical artery dissection struggle with chronic fatigue. What may seem like simple physical activities can lead to exhaustion. Social activities associated with noise and overstimulation can be difficult. Stressful situations can also increase exhaustion. Sleep quality and duration can also be poor following a brain injury, but some patients with carotid and vertebral artery dissections experience difficulty sleeping even when a stroke has not resulted from the vascular injury, which can lead to both fatigue and difficulty with pain management.

Our brains are wired for us to sleep at night. When light vanishes from the environment, a hormone called melatonin is produced by the pineal gland in the brain, which helps to regulate the circadian rhythms involved in our sleep cycles. When light returns, melatonin production decreases. Adequate, restful sleep is a critical part of pain management and dissection recovery. If a patient is not sleeping and has refractory migraines, one of the first goals should be to get the sleep disturbance under control. It makes no sense to load a patient on medications for pain if helping him/her to sleep better will achieve a significant reduction in pain and fatigue.

Following a carotid or vertebral dissection patients can have difficulty regulating circadian rhythms and may need assistance. Caffeine elimination, avoiding excessive fluid intake before bed, adhering to a regular bedtime routine, going to sleep at a time that will allow for 7-8 hours of sleep during dark hours – all of these are necessary considerations. Working night shifts makes treating fatigue and pain nearly impossible in the stroke population. Those who are experiencing fatigue or pain after a cervical artery dissection with or without stroke who work overnight should consider inquiring about switching to a shift that takes place during daylight hours. If these changes do not work to yield a full night of restful sleep reliably, sleep medications may be utilized. They all have the potential for side effects, so sleep medications should be individualized based on each patient's history and symptoms. If a stroke patient cannot sleep because of extreme anxiety, for example, then a benzodiazepine (medication that can be used for sleep and for anxiety) might be chosen, although these have the potential for dependence. If a stroke patient does not sleep well and has refractory pain, the pain is unlikely to be controlled until the sleep issue is addressed.

Although there is a lack of research specific to cervical artery dissection and fatigue, the National Stroke Association reports that up to 70% of stroke survivors suffer from fatigue.

Fatigue after a carotid or vertebral artery dissection is very different than simply feeling tired. Fatigue after a cervical artery dissection can be one of the most debilitating invisible symptoms associated with this injury. It doesn't necessarily improve with rest, and can result from not only physical activities, but from sensory overload, emotional distress, and from tasks like reading that require concentration.[141] Unfortunately, the fatigue that occurs after stroke and cervical dissection can last for many years.

There is no specific medication that can combat fatigue, but there are some lifestyle adjustments that can be made to help. The National Stroke Association recommends that you share with your family and friends how you are feeling. Don't be afraid to speak up and let everyone know if you are feeling fatigued. Sometimes it is a matter of too many stimuli coming in at once. If your closest support network is aware of the situations that are the most difficult for you, it will be much easier to take regular rest breaks without feeling the need to explain yourself each time.

The National Stroke Association also recommends keeping a journal of your daily activities and how you feel. A healthy diet full of fruits and vegetables can improve your energy level. Be careful not to limit calories too much on an extreme diet, which can decrease your energy level and lead to hypoglycemia and headaches.

A light to moderate exercise program also can improve energy levels. Be aware of your limits, though. Keep a journal of your exercise and how your energy level is impacted. You may be tempted to add an intense exercise program to your regimen, but give yourself time and gradually build up your exercise intensity.

"Why am I having trouble concentrating and remembering things ever since my dissection?"

Patients who have experienced a carotid or vertebral artery dissection with or without a resulting stroke frequently notice impaired focus and concentration. Although there are many survivor accounts reporting exhaustion after a dissection, there is very limited research documenting the long-term effects of vertebral and carotid artery dissections. There are, however, multiple studies linking brain injury and stroke to chronic fatigue. Research has linked brain injury to long-term fatigue, malaise, dizziness and mild cognitive impairment.[142] In a study of young patients (ages 18 to 50) with either TIA or stroke, 41% experienced symptoms of impaired concentration and problem solving.[143]

It is well-documented that patients battling chronic pain have challenges with focus and concentration. Because cervical artery dissection patients frequently have concurrent issues with pain, it should not be surprising that they experience some cognitive impairments even when no known brain injury has occurred.

"I didn't have a stroke but I'm having memory problems, concentration problems, and fatigue. Is it possible I had brain damage that doesn't show up on scans?"

Cognitive changes after a carotid or vertebral artery dissection can be very real, even if there is no evidence of stroke present on a brain MRI. There are several reasons why this may be the case.

The average adult brain contains over 80 *billion* neurons, and current neurological diagnostic technology is not powerful enough to detect whether there is damage present in every cell. Microinfarcts can cause cognitive impairments but go undetected by imaging scans.[144]

There have been research studies examining microinfarcts related to dementia and traumatic brain injury. Sometimes brain damage is only visible during an autopsy and microscopic examination of brain tissue. More research is needed to better understand the presence of microinfarcts in the setting of carotid or vertebral artery dissection, but it is entirely possible there is damaged brain tissue causing impairments that CT scans and MRIs are not revealing.

Additionally, if an MRI is obtained too early into an ischemic stroke, it is possible that a small stroke was present, but is not yet evident on the scan, which is particularly true in the brainstem territory, where evidence of ischemia can be delayed.

Cognitive symptoms are very common in patients suffering from refractory migraines. Even if there is not an injury to the brain, such as what occurs with stroke, impaired memory and focus may be present because a person is stuck in a migrainous state that is unrelenting. The same is true with sleep deprivation. If insomnia is part of dissection aftermath, even if a stroke is not present, it is difficult to retain new information and perform at a high level in this sleep-deprived state.

Chapter 14: Patient story

Finding Support

In 2008, I was a very fit, healthy 39-year-old married man with two young children. I had been looking for a challenge and decided to represent Citi, playing badminton, in the London Corporate Games in October. In the six weeks leading up to the games, I stepped up my training, shed the last few unwanted couple of pounds, and felt in good shape. On the Saturday of the games, I qualified for the knockout stages of the men's singles and doubles. On Sunday, I won the quarter and semifinals of the singles before preparing for the semifinals.

It was while I warmed up for that match that I experienced what I now know were the first symptoms of my dissected carotid artery. Suddenly, the middle two fingers on my right hand stopped working and wouldn't let go of the racket. After a few seconds my fingers released, and I carried on, but it happened again about six times in the next five minutes. I thought it must be a spasm in my tendon and carried on playing. I was also aware during that game that my sense of direction while smashing the shuttle was well off of normal; never mind, I thought, as my partner and I went on to win the match. When I came off of the court, I had the strongest urge to eat chocolate that I've ever had (I don't eat it often) but the café had sold out.

Somehow, I managed to win the singles and doubles finals and headed off home via the M25 feeling somewhat exhausted. I felt lethargic and had no sense of urgency. I was happy to drive home slowly, which was unusual for me. On Sunday evening, I went to bed early. On Monday at lunchtime, I headed to the office gym as usual, but I had no energy or motivation to do anything. After 10 minutes, I got changed and went back to my desk. I'd never felt like that before. Tuesday, it was exactly the same experience, and I began to feel frustrated. Things were going to change on Wednesday, I told myself, so I joined a spin class in the afternoon, in the hope that would motivate me, which it did.

I now realize my body was telling me to slow down as it tried to heal the artery I had dissected, and I should have listened. During the warm down session, at the end of the class, my middle two right fingers started to tingle, like pins and needles, and then my left eyeball started throbbing, which was immediately followed by an acute stabbing pain that felt like someone was repeatedly jabbing a red, hot poker in my ear. I dismounted the bike and felt a little wobbly, however, I managed to get to the changing room and get showered. Across the busy changing room, I tried to tell the instructor what had happened to me, but the words I wanted to say wouldn't come out of my mouth properly - odd. I tried again, but I couldn't seem to speak properly. I headed back to my desk, sat down and logged onto my computer. I clicked to open an e-mail. On the screen in front of me was a normal e-mail; the only difference was that I couldn't understand it - any of it. I knew that there were words, I knew it was a sentence, and I knew I should be able to read it, but I couldn't. I turned to tell a colleague; again, I was unable to get the words out of my mouth, even though I knew exactly what I wanted to say. At that point, I started to lose vision in my left eye. Everything went pixelates with bright white spots.

While I sat quietly, waiting for home time, my symptoms subsided, and my wife called me. I explained what had happened, and she said that I still sounded funny. I agreed to meet her on the way home. I met my wife at the station, and she took me immediately to the doctor. I was admitted to the Medical Emergency Ward of the local hospital that afternoon, where I stayed for nearly two weeks. In total, I experienced seven transient ischemic attacks (TIAs) in a four-week period, each with slightly different symptoms, including paralysis, loss of speech, drooping face, vision loss and many more. An MRI scan in the hospital identified a carotid artery dissection as the cause of my TIAs. It took six months to heal. I returned to work full-time in June 2009.

During my time in the hospital, my wife found it very difficult to find information about dissections or the prognosis for my future. At one point, she was advised to prepare for me not making it. That sense of frustration my wife experienced is what gave me the idea of creating a support group on Facebook. I had already been at home resting for a couple of months and was looking for things to pass the time of day. I had only recently joined Facebook, so I thought I'd see how to create a group.

I never actually expected anyone to find it or join, as it was just a way for me to collate some information and learn how to build a group. I created lots of different discussion threads based on all the questions I wanted answered and, once finished, didn't think much more about it. A few weeks later, someone joined and started adding comments on my discussion threads. Then a few more joined over the coming weeks. Some of these initial members I added as personal friends on Facebook. Over the coming months, the numbers gradually increased, and I created a spreadsheet to record where people were located, how old they were when they dissected, etc. Within six months, we were approaching 100 members. I stopped adding members in my spreadsheet.

As the group grew in size, some members asked

for the group to become 'closed' so their own friends could not see any posts they made. I continue to keep the group 'open' so that anyone can find the group and read the posts, at any time, from anywhere. They just need to search on Facebook for carotid artery dissection and the group will show up. The way I look at it, if someone had a dissection today and their partner/family wanted to understand more about dissections, the information is readily available. Access to this information is really important and shouldn't be hidden.

Common themes began to appear within the group. Most members were approximately 35-45 years of age when it happened and were extremely fit and active prior to their dissections. Symptoms mainly fell into two groups: TIA/stroke-related or Horner syndrome. For most of us, we'll never know the cause of our dissections. Some have been able to identify genetic causes (i.e. fibromuscular dysplasia), and others have been induced 'trauma' related events. One was caused during learning how to use the flying trapeze, and another was caused by head-banging at a 40th birthday party! The members of the group now cover the globe, and I've been fortunate enough to meet a few over the years. Six of us met up in London and on two separate occasions, I have met families from the US, when they have been in London on holiday, and we've had lunch and shown them around.

I am now approaching eight years since my dissection and consider myself very fortunate to have made a significant recovery. People meeting me would never know what had happened to me, but my close family notice the small details that have changed post-dissection.

Our group, as of 2017, has in excess of 1,550 members and increases on a weekly basis.

Chapter 15:

Life After Dissection

"I feel so different on the inside since my carotid dissection, but I look like my old self to everyone else. How do I get others to understand that I am not able to handle everything I used to do?"

One of the most common frustrations that patients with cervical artery dissections express is that because they look so "normal" to others, the expectation is that nothing has changed. However, they frequently have ongoing symptoms or feel different. There is guilt. Patients state something along the lines of: "I know how lucky I am, because it could have been so much worse, but I still don't feel well. Others expect me to just be everything I was before because I do look the same and don't have obvious deficits."

After a cervical artery dissection, it is especially important to pace yourself and make sure you get plenty of rest. Don't be afraid to say no to others and put your health first. Be honest about how you are feeling, and communicate with your family about what you can and can't do. It is unrealistic to expect yourself to jump right back into your old life. It takes time to heal.

This book is an ideal resource to share with family members to help explain your health issues. Also, you may want to encourage family members and friends to join online support groups for dissection survivors so they can read about what others are experiencing.

When others are empathetic and want to be supportive, this is huge. Holidays and travel can be especially taxing. When people offer to help you, take them up on it! You will need to build a support system of understanding friends and family.

"I've heard from a few healthcare providers that my symptoms are not related to my dissection and I am just dealing with stress and anxiety. Am I crazy?"

No, you are not! Symptoms of fatigue, pain, anxiety, memory difficulty, and problems with concentration can certainly result from cervical artery dissections. Survivors commonly experience these symptoms. Individuals with cervical artery dissections have found great comfort from learning that they are not alone in their struggles.

Unfortunately, there is not a lot of recognition in the general medical community about lingering symptoms following this vascular injury. Patients can find themselves frustrated when their symptoms do not resolve, but the artery appears to have healed on follow-up radiological studies. Remember the analogy from earlier about a skin wound: it may "heal," but it frequently is not the same as the original intact skin that used to be there.

"Ever since my vertebral artery dissection, I've been so dizzy. When I tilt my head the room starts spinning. When should I be concerned about this dizziness, and what can I do about it?"

Vertigo can be a beast of a symptom to endure. After all, if Alfred Hitchcock named a movie after a neurological symptom, then it must be extremely unpleasant to experience. Vertigo refers to the perception of movement when there is no movement taking place. For some, this means having the sensation of the room spinning around them. It may be impossible to stand upright because of the lack of orientation. Others may feel as though they are walking on a boat that is wavering back and forth.

Vertigo, in particular, may be a symptom of a vertebral artery dissection, as the vertebral arteries supply blood to the cerebellum, which is the balance and coordination command center for the brain. However, vertigo is a common symptom of migraine as well. Anyone with a brain injury who develops migraines as a complication of that injury may begin to see vertigo rearing its ugly head.

Unfortunately, vertigo can be present for years after a stroke, and some patients with vertebral artery dissections continuing to experience it even when a stroke has not been confirmed on a brain MRI. If associated with other symptoms of migraine, it is worth focusing on migraine management in order to alleviate the vertigo (see chapter 11 on migraine management). If vertigo does not seem to be associated with migraine, desensitization exercises with a trained physical therapist can be helpful. Meclizine is a medication that can be used to treat this sort of dizziness as needed. When not effective, certain benzodiazepines can also be used, such as diazepam (Valium), lorazepam (Ativan), or clonazepam (Klonapin), but keep in mind that these medications can cause dependence or addiction, so it will be important to weigh the risks and the benefits of these.

"Since my dissection and stroke, I have continued to have problems with swallowing. What can I do about this?"

If you continue to have difficulty swallowing (dysphagia) after your dissection and/or stroke, a speech-language pathologist can address this issue. When you are evaluated by a speech therapist, you will likely be given a set of specific exercises and compensatory strategies to help you swallow. You may temporarily need to drink thickened liquids and to avoid certain foods until your swallowing function improves if you are found to have dysphagia.

Swallowing impairments vary from one patient to another, so there is no one-size-fits-all treatment approach. Your speech therapist may request an order from your doctor for a modified barium swallow study. A modified barium swallow study will provide your Speech-Language Pathologist with extremely helpful information that will guide your treatment plan.

For more information about dysphagia visit www.asha.org.

"Sometimes my hands and feet get numb. Does this mean I'm having a TIA?"

Following cervical artery dissections, a substantial number of patients who are battling chronic headaches will mention numbness and/or tingling in their hands and feet as a concern. The first question a physician should ask is whether they are taking topiramate (Topamax) for migraine management. Topamax is an anti-seizure medication that is also widely used for reducing the intensity and frequency of migraine attacks. Patients are often unaware that a common side effect of this medication is numbness and tingling in the hands and feet. It is usually benign, and if the tingling is too bothersome, your physician may recommend stopping the drug.

Hyperventilation is another potential origin of numbness and tingling in the hands and feet. People who are experiencing significant anxiety frequently hyperventilate without even recognizing it. More frequent breathing results in blowing off more carbon dioxide, which affects the pH of a person's blood, may cause tingling in the hands and feet.

Peripheral neuropathy (nerve damage) is a common cause of this symptom, but this reaction is usually more gradual (over months to years) rather than coming on more quickly (over days to weeks). Causes of neuropathy include diabetes mellitus, excessive alcohol use, genetic disorders, and exposure to certain heavy metals, to name a few.

Numbness in both hands and both feet is not typically reflective of a TIA, unless the brainstem is involved. However, numbness and tingling affecting an arm and a leg on one side of the body (and especially if the face is also involved) is more cause for concern and should be evaluated immediately in an emergency department if the onset is sudden.

"I'm getting mixed information about what activities I can do. I have been given a variety of restrictions after my dissection? Can I lift heavy objects? Can I work out?"

Survivors also wonder what types of activities are safe after a cervical artery dissection. It is difficult to provide all-inclusive advice on what to avoid and what is likely safe, because life is filled with infinite possibilities. In general, it is advised that patients who have sustained carotid or vertebral artery dissections avoid activities that would be likely to result in trauma to the neck. Some neurologists recommend against riding roller-coasters, undergoing cervical spine manipulations, or participating in extreme forms of exercise during which the neck is stretched and twisted. If coughing led to the dissection, it may be worth using cough suppressant interventions (honey, medications) early to avoid prolonged severe coughing spells. If the dissection occurred while straining during a bowel movement, using a stool softener during periods of constipation makes intuitive sense.

"How much weight can I safely lift, especially now that my dissection has healed on my follow up scans?"

Unfortunately, there is not a simple answer to this question. A well-conditioned individual who has been weightlifting for years may lift 70 pounds easily and without straining to do so, while another person may have to strain to lift a 20-pound grocery bag. The key is to avoid extreme straining. If you're having to bear down and strain to lift a load, then it is probably too heavy for someone who has dissected an artery.

Also remember that if the dissection occurred because you were in a car accident, that presents a much lower risk for spontaneous dissections going forward than in someone who experienced a dissection from a mild inciting action, such as sneezing or coughing (or not even knowing what caused it). If your dissection occurred because of a severe whiplash injury when you were rear-ended by a vehicle, many people with healthy blood vessels probably would have ended up with a dissection under such circumstances. Straining a little during a weightlifting activity is probably not going to present a substantial risk for spontaneous dissection once the vessel has healed.

"Can I fly on an airplane, six months after my carotid dissection occurred?"

Patients frequently ask about whether a pressurized cabin on a plane can pose risk to them after a carotid or vertebral artery dissection. There is no evidence that flying on a plane after a dissection, especially once the artery is no longer acutely injured, poses significant risk of harm.

Consider this: car crashes are much more common than airplane collisions. Therefore, since carotid and vertebral artery dissections are not uncommon after car accidents, perhaps the airplane is the safer option for travel in this patient group!

"I'm worried about my health and providing for my family. Is it possible to get a life insurance policy with a medical history of a carotid or vertebral artery dissection?"

Life insurance can be tricky after any major medical event, including dissections. If you were not insured before the event, and now you want life insurance coverage, there is little you can do other than apply for coverage and see what happens. If your dissection was caused by a traumatic event, such as a car accident, then you can explain this detail on the application, and that may not preclude you from becoming insured. Some policies have a blackout period for three years or five years after an event, so if you are denied on the first attempt, it is worth reapplying later if this is the case.

"I really want to have kids. Is it safe to get pregnant after a dissection?"

There is no definitive evidence to make definitive recommendations here, but wanting to have a baby is certainly a natural instinct for most women. It is possible that removing the straining, bearing down, and pushing from delivery by choosing a cesarean delivery ("C-section") may be a safer option in a patient who has had a cervical artery dissection. There is always the possibility of surgical complications by going the C-section route, and these risks should be discussed with your healthcare provider. Make sure your provider understands your health history and has gone over the possible complications during pregnancy and delivery with you. It is also worth discussing pregnancy with your neurologist and getting his or her opinion.

Know that *many* women with a history of carotid or vertebral artery dissection later go through pregnancy and delivery without complications and do very well. Do not assume that the answer to the question of whether you should pursue a dream of having children is "no" because of a dissection in your past. Surround yourself by a good team of healthcare professionals with expertise in this area and have an honest conversation.

"Nobody seems to understand what I am going through. How can I find a support group?"

Social media has had a wonderful impact on the lives of people who are struggling to cope with carotid and vertebral dissections. Online support groups are an excellent way to find other survivors who understand what you are experiencing.

There are multiple support groups that you can join on Facebook specifically for dissection survivors Facebook is a great place to connect with other survivors and share experiences. However, avoid seeking medical advice and always discuss issues with your medical provider before making any changes to your plan of care.

"How long should I wait before I return to work after my dissection?"

You may need additional time off from your job before you return after a cervical artery dissection. If you have sick leave and/or short-term disability benefits, this can be very helpful as you take the time to recover.

The question about timing the return to work is unique to each individual, and it partially depends on the type of work that you do, the severity of the dissection, whether a stroke occurred, and many other factors. Some patients do not have any symptoms of their dissection a week later and go on to lead normal lives. Others struggle for years with symptoms.

"I want to work, but I am in so much pain, and I am exhausted all the time. I can't perform my old job, or any job for that matter. Is it possible to get disability benefits?"

Some of the topics neurologists spend the most time discussing with patients and their families who are facing the aftermath of dissection have nothing to do with actual medicine. When physicians enter the world of clinical practice, while patients depend on them to guide them in making decisions that impact their health, they also want to answers that physicians are not formally trained to answer. The non-medical topic that may be discussed the most frequently with stroke and dissection patients is the process of applying for disability income.

The first time a patient asked me why she was turned down for social security, I had no idea. She clearly was physically disabled from her stroke. I had completed the appropriate paperwork sent to my office. I could see she was visibly upset at being denied this needed income, and I felt guilty, as if it was my fault in some way, despite my having meticulously completed the forms. What happened?

Over time I have gained more insight into why this scenario occurs. My disclaimer here is that I am not an attorney, employed by the federal government, or a certified account, so what I am sharing is purely what I have gained from watching hundreds of stroke patients navigate the process. Patients frequently do not understand how the system works, and many healthcare providers don't either. To be perfectly frank, I am naïve to all of the inner-workings of "the system," but I can boil it down to a few key points that I hope will provide clarity to anyone out there living with neurological deficits after stroke.

Stroke patients in the United States essentially have two options available for long term disability income: private disability insurance and/or social security.

If a long term disability insurance policy was purchased prior to the stroke from a company such as The Hartford, MetLife, or Liberty Mutual (these are only a handful of carriers out of the many available), then a claim can be filed. The patient's healthcare provider, usually a physician, will be asked to complete paperwork, and copies of relevant medical records will be requested and sent.

Typically, there is a waiting period, which is variable. If a patient has short-term disability insurance, income from that policy can be used for part or all of the waiting period until the long- term disability income is available. If there is no short-term disability policy in place and no sick leave available, there is usually a lengthy unpaid period as the patient waits. If a patient improves over the course of the waiting period, even if a long term disability policy is present, the patient may not be eligible to receive income if the level of disability cannot be verified in the medical records or from the paperwork completed by the healthcare provider.

Then, there is Social Security, which is one of the most misunderstood systems in the U.S. Patients have so many different ideas of what social security is, how it works, how one receives benefits, and so on. The National Stroke Association does a fantastic job of breaking down Social Security on its website. Visit www.stroke.org and write *disability* in the search bar to reach the information regarding applying for Social Security disability benefits.

In the example I mentioned above, the reason the patient was denied social security income was not because she was not physically disabled, but because her stroke was less than one year old. Her stroke was too recent. The condition has to be expected to last "at least

12 months." Then, I have seen patients who are approved less than 12 months from the time of the event. My advice to stroke patients who have been denied Social Security income if they applied less than one year after the stroke is to re-apply after a year has passed.

If a patient is already receiving Social Security income because of his or her age (let's say – a 70-year-old patient who has been receiving Social Security income for five years), then the patient is already receiving the money. People do not receive double the amount of money for becoming disabled over the age at which they become eligible to receive social security income. If an adult has never worked, or worked but somehow never paid into the program, or if a person worked but did not contribute enough to the program while working, then a person is probably not eligible to receive Social Security income.

If there are questions about your personal situation, contact an attorney with expertise in this area. It's important for patients to understand that Social Security is an annuity, meaning that people pay into the program as an insurance policy. In return, money is paid out, either when a person becomes disabled or when a person reaches retirement age.

Social Security defines disability based on your ability to work. You are considered disabled by social security if you cannot do the work that you did before, if they decide they you can't adjust to other work because of your medical condition, and your disability has lasted at least one year or will result in death.[145] For those who had a dissection with no overt physical impairments but pain and fatigue it could be more challenging to get approval for disability benefits. Again, consulting with an attorney who has expertise in this area is recommended if this is presenting problems for you.

"Is it safe to drive after a carotid or vertebral artery dissection?"

If you have experienced any visual symptoms as a result of your dissection, you need to schedule an appointment with an ophthalmologist or optometrist to have your vision assessed before you start to drive. If a stroke has occurred, sometimes there can be loss of vision in a visual field (homonymous hemianopia if half of a visual field is missing - please see page 58 on visual abnormalities for more details). It can be difficult for patients to recognize the degree of visual impairment they may have in this scenario, but an opthamologist or optometrist can perform visual field testing to test for this condition. Patients with carotid artery dissections can also experience "strokes in the eye," meaning a blood clot can travel to one of the arteries supplying blood flow to the retina or optic nerve and visual loss can occur. Obviously, driving with a significant visual impairment poses a risk to your safety as well as to that of others, so a visual assessment and clearance from one of these trained eyecare professional is imperative.

Patients may also have cognitive deficits, in particular if stroke has occurred as a result of the dissection. They can have difficulty focusing and concentrating. They may feel excessively tired, and fall asleep easily, even in the midst of activity. All of these should be red flags for returning right away to driving and should be discussed with a healthcare professional beforehand. If there is uncertainty about a patient's cognitive ability to drive, such as whether a driver would be able to react and stop in time if a person suddenly ran in front of the car. Some occupational therapists are trained to perform driving evaluations, and they can provide recommendations about readiness to drive. Patients frequently ask their neurologists for a definitive recommendation about returning to driving in this setting. If a person has obvious cognitive limitations, it is an easier question to answer, but if deficits are subtle, since a neurologist is not going to be riding in the car with a patient, there is often not a clear answer. With an occupational therapist, a detailed assessment can be performed and frequently a driving simulation to measure reaction times to real world situations on the road.

Adaptations may have to be made to your vehicle. A new vehicle already adapted for the disabled can be purchased if there are new physical limitations as the result of stroke, such as weakness in the right leg.

Once given the all clear to start driving again, take extra care when checking your blind spots and merging. Turn your neck slowly and use your mirrors as much as possible. Make sure your seatbelt does not rest on your neck. You can purchase seat belt adjuster straps to achieve a proper fit across your chest and shoulder.

If driving is proving to cause you large amounts of stress, then allow for more time before pursuing it. Driving can prove very challenging for patients in less populated areas where public transportation is limited or nonexistent to continue with their daily lives while not driving.

"I don't want to become a hypochondriac, but when is it important to seek immediate medical attention? Every new symptom I have has me thinking I am dissecting again or having a stroke."

Your new normal will be finding a balance between realistic concerns for protecting yourself from another dissection, living with the symptoms and participating in your normal life as much as possible.

Because carotid and/or vertebral artery dissections catches patients off guard, there is a level of vulnerability that accompanies this vascular injury, and with vulnerability comes fear. The safe answer for everyone when a patient calls with a new concern is to go to the emergency department. However, many would argue that life cannot be lived in an emergency department. So how does a fearful individual learn to recognize which symptoms are concerning and which ones are not?

In general, new symptoms that could be consistent with stroke need to be addressed urgently in the emergency department. These include, but are not limited to: slurred speech, sudden difficulty walking (due to impaired balance or new weakness), numbness/tingling in your arm and/or leg, suddenly impaired vision, sudden onset of weakness in an arm and/or leg, sudden onset of drooping on one side of the face, and difficulty speaking and/or understanding language.

Familiarize yourself with the signs and symptoms for stroke. You can quickly screen yourself or someone near you for signs of stroke by using the acronym FAST:

- **Face:** If you are worried that you may be having a stroke, check your face in the mirror. Smile and see if one side of your face is drooping.

- **Arms:** Try raising your arms in front of you, and make sure you can hold them up. If one arm drifts downward this may indicate that a stroke is occurring.
- **Speech:** If you are alone, try saying aloud a familiar phrase like: "It's raining cats and dogs." If your speech is slurred or if you are unable to produce the words entirely, this is concerning for stroke until proven otherwise. In some cases, you may not be able to recognize any deficits even if they exist because of damage to receptive language portion of your brain, so if you are uncertain and another person is available, try to talk to him or her.
- **Time:** If you or another person are showing any of the mentioned signs of stroke, it is important that 911 be called if you are in the United States, or the appropriate emergency response number for your area if you are outside of the United States.

With a history of carotid or vertebral artery dissection with or without stroke, preparing a medical history form ahead of time to give to the medical staff in the emergency department helps to expedite care. The sheet should include your medical history, an up-to-date list of your medications (including doses you are taking, as well as how frequently the medication is taken), your medication allergies, and anything else you would want your healthcare professionals to know if you are unable to communicate with them.

What about for other symptoms that may not necessarily indicate that a stroke is occurring? Unfortunately, there is not a simple answer to this question. A good relationship with a neurologist is important, so that when you have concerns about a symptom that may be less urgent, he or she can guide you on whether further imaging should be performed, medications should be changed, or whether a trip to the emergency department is recommended. Every situation is unique. If headaches are worsening, but a patient recently stopped a migraine preventative medication, that likely will not warrant a trip to the emergency department. If neck pain is more severe, but a patient is already on optimal medical therapy to present stroke and no stroke symptoms are present, a neurologist may opt to repeat a CT-angiogram or MR-angiogram in the outpatient setting rather than sending someone to the emergency department since a change in management is unlikely.

When in doubt, though, presenting to the emergency department is a good idea.

"Going to the ER is so expensive. Can I just go to urgent care if I am having new symptoms?"

No! Urgent care clinics provide a needed, useful service in providing care for patients who either lack primary care providers or whose primary care offices are closed. A routine sinus infection or urinary tract infection can usually be treated at an urgent care clinic. Complex vascular injuries cannot. For starters, the vast majority of urgent care clinics will not have CT or MRI scanners, and if you have had a carotid or vertebral artery dissection and are now presenting with symptoms concerning for stroke, the urgent care provider is going to have to send you to the emergency department anyway for imaging. The additional trip to urgent care before the emergency department creates a delay in your treatment.

Many hospitals now are certified by the Joint Commission as "Primary Stroke Centers," which means they have met quality metrics and have demonstrated readiness to rapidly and appropriately deliver care to patients with acute strokes. There is no such process for urgent care clinics and stroke certification.

Additionally, urgent care clinics do not have IV t-PA available to administer, so if you are a candidate for this drug and go to an urgent care clinic, you will then be sent on to the emergency department. Again, the trip to the urgent care clinic creates a delay in treatment, and with delays come worse outcomes over the long term.

Stroke is a serious problem, and patients can look very well one minute, and the next minute become very unstable, requiring urgent medical intervention.

The bottom line: if you have a carotid or vertebral dissection and have new concerning symptoms, especially those described in the previous section, the right call to make is 911.

"When I had my dissection, I sat in the waiting room at the ER for hours before I was seen. I'm terrified of having another dissection or a stroke and having the staff at the ER ignore me. Is there anything I can do so I can get immediate medical attention?"

This is another reason to call 911 if an individual is having new symptoms concerning for stroke. When a patient arrives by ambulance, he or she is almost always brought directly back to be evaluated by healthcare providers upon arrival.

Emergency departments have triage systems in place to help determine which patients should be seen urgently and which ones are able to wait in favor of caring for the most emergent cases. While healthcare providers strive to correctly identify urgent needs, the system is not perfect. However, if your concern is for stroke, and you feel you need to be evaluated urgently, if you tell the triage provider, "I think I am having a stroke," that usually gets things moving quickly.

If you are in the United States, it is also helpful to know which hospitals in your area are certified as Primary Stroke Centers. In urban areas, there is usually at least one. More rural hospitals are becoming certified, but there are still many areas where this is not the case. Larger hospitals and academic medical centers are Comprehensive Stroke Centers, which carry higher certification. This certification means that the facilities are equipped with all of the possible specialists, equipment, and facilities to care for any potential stroke type or stroke complication that presents Primary and Comprehensive Stroke Centers have to report the number of strokes they treat each year and track data on the quality of stroke care being delivered. Again, while nothing is perfect, these stroke centers may be more likely to detect strokes at presentation and have a system in place for rapidly evaluating these patients.

"I take more medications than my 90-year-old grandmother. The people who work at the pharmacy look at me like I'm nuts. Is there anything I can do?"

Because carotid and vertebral artery dissection patients are usually young, healthy adults, it can be a jolt to them to suddenly be taking multiple medications. Because preventing stroke and controlling symptoms of headaches, neck pain, muscle spasm, sleep disturbances, and/or anxiety are all part of the aftermath, a person who has never taken medications may find himself or herself on six or seven of them, or perhaps even more.

It is a good idea to get to know your pharmacist and to fill prescriptions consistently at the same pharmacy if you have a place you know and trust. You do not need to necessarily explain your situation, but since sometimes dissection survivors can appear so normal physically, it might be a good idea to take a minute and talk to your pharmacist about your prescriptions if you are concerned about being misunderstood and ask questions if you have them.

Pharmacists are the unsung heroes of healthcare and provide critically important services as part of a care team, even though they are often working behind the scenes. Engaging pharmacists as part of your healthcare team will lead to more comfort on your part and understanding of your needs on the other side. In particular, if you have been prescribed controlled substances, such as opioids for pain or benzodiazepines for anxiety, it may make you feel more at ease to explain your diagnosis to your pharmacist.

"Is it safe to smoke after a dissection?"

Dissection or no dissection - smoking is not safe. Whether you have had a dissection or not, smoking still places you at risk for cancers, heart attacks, and strokes, to name a few concerns.

Since quitting is so important, ask your doctor for help. Join support groups and commit to stop smoking. Addiction is a powerful thing, and quitting can be an extremely challenging process. Most people who attempt to quit will start smoking again multiple times before they are finally successful. The key is not to give up. If you try to quit, are successful for a month, and then return to smoking - okay, that is a month where you were successful. The next time around hopefully it will be longer. Focus on one day at a time and stay in the present when you are attempting to quit, rather than feeling overwhelmed by the long term. Celebrate your milestones and reward yourself. Do what you need to do to quit.

"Is it okay to drink alcoholic beverages after a dissection?"

In general, an occasional alcoholic drink will not harm most people, whether they have had a cervical artery dissection or not. Everything in moderation, right? However, other factors have to be considered. Patients who have other conditions that make alcohol more dangerous (such as liver disease) should avoid it.

There is no literature published demonstrating that alcohol is any more harmful to people who have had dissections than it is for the general population. That being said, if patients start medications to control symptoms after dissection, then this has to be considered when making decisions about alcohol consumption. The breakdown process of medications that are metabolized by the liver can be disrupted (either sped up or slowed down) in the presence of alcohol, since alcohol is also metabolized by the liver. It may also take less alcohol than usual to intoxicate a person if these sorts of medications are present. Use caution and discuss the use of alcohol with your healthcare provider.

"When, if ever, will I start to feel better?"

This question comes up repeatedly, and sadly is not addressed in any available resources for patients with carotid or vertebral artery dissections. Many survivors are frequently provided with very little information about what life will be like in the months, and potentially years, ahead.

Every situation is unique. Some patients never experience bothersome symptoms and only end up diagnosed because a family member notices that the pupils are different sizes. Others live in agonizing refractory pain for years following a dissection. Therefore, giving specific information about when a patient will start to feel better is challenging. However, here is what can be said:

- There is no "normal" that applies to everyone with a carotid or vertebral artery dissection. Many patients feel better within several weeks of a dissection. However, many do not.
- Just because arteries look normal once more on a CT-angiogram or an MR-angiogram, months after a dissection does not mean that all symptoms should be gone. Think about it. If you have a major traumatic abdominal injury from a terrible car accident, just because a follow-up scan months later may then look normal, pain can still exist.
- You will likely feel better if you are sleeping regularly and for a prolonged enough period of time each night. Sleep disturbances make pain and anxiety difficult to treat. If symptoms are unrelenting months after a dissection, evaluate your sleep quality and duration to see if this could be contributing.
- If you are still miserable months later and have been resistant to the idea of using medications to

manage symptoms, know that some patients only need medications to get symptoms under control and then wean off of them later. It's not a certainty that if you use a medication like a migraine preventative agent for a few months to get your headaches under control that you will still be using it five years later. However, sometimes medication is needed to at least gain better control of the problem, at least initially.

"Is it safe to have sex after a carotid or vertebral artery dissection?"

This topic has also not been definitively studied, but it is an important quality-of-life question for most patients. As with all physical activity after dissection, use moderation and pace yourself when returning to it. Many neurologists will recommend that patients hold off on having sex for at least a few weeks after a recent dissection to exercise caution. Overexertion during sexual activity has been reported in the literature as causing carotid and vertebral dissections in certain cases, but then again, so has straining during a bowel movement - and we are not going to recommend that you stop having bowel movements.[146]

If you are concerned about another vascular injury during sex, and it is affecting your relationship, have an honest conversation with your partner about it. Be careful with positioning your neck and be mindful of the amount of straining involved.

"What can I do to help raise awareness about dissections?"

For some, the feeling of vulnerability from a carotid or vertebral artery dissection can cause patients to become hesitant about discussing their experiences, and prefer to remain private. Others want to share their stories openly in hopes that the condition will become more recognized. Both approaches are okay, and no one should feel pressured to discuss something personal if there is discomfort with doing so.

If you are comfortable sharing your story, then this is probably the best way to raise awareness. Simply allowing people who know you to associate a familiar person with this vascular injury and/or stroke. Since dissection patients are usually young, if you have had a stroke and feel ready to share that, then it also raises awareness that stroke can occur at any age.

You may want to write a letter to the hospital that treated you to say thank you if you believe your care was good or to give feedback if the diagnosis was initially missed. If the latter is the case, then explain that you are interested in helping to improve the institution's ability to properly diagnose individuals with carotid or vertebral artery dissection, and would be happy to discuss your experience further. Personal stories can go a long way towards building awareness, and with awareness comes more prompt diagnosis and treatment when dissections occur in the future.

"I want to participate in a research study, but I don't know where to start. What sort of research is being done on cervical artery dissections?"

Surprisingly, there are many studies devoted to carotid and vertebral artery dissections. To see those that have been published already, you can search for "carotid dissection" or "vertebral dissection" at http://pubmed.gov. Unfortunately, there is a dearth of information about the aftermath once the acute stage has ended. At any point in time in the United States, if you are seeking an actively recruiting study to join, you can search for those same terms at http://www.clinicaltrials.gov.

Afterword

Carotid and vertebral artery dissections are not rare occurrences, although many healthcare providers have this impression. The majority of patients who are diagnosed with these vascular injuries are completely unfamiliar with the term. Since the symptoms associated with carotid and vertebral artery dissections are so similar to other, more common medical ailments such as migraine or muscular spasm, that diagnosis is often delayed or not made at all. We believe they are underdiagnosed.

It is important to accurately diagnose these patients, because failing to start appropriate therapy can result in stroke that might have otherwise been prevented. One of the main reasons we wrote this book was to raise awareness about the early presentation of carotid and vertebral artery dissections in hopes that it would become more recognized in mainstream life.

Perhaps the largest driving force pushing us to create this resource for patients and their loved ones was to give those impacted by this diagnosis a starting place for understanding the problem and hopefully to provide insight into some of its aftermath. Over the years, we have heard many dissection survivors wonder why they may still have symptoms long after their vascular injuries because they were under the impression that the symptoms should be short-lived, which is a common misconception. We wanted to let patients know that having symptoms months and even years later can be *normal* in this setting.

Given that these patients are young, healthy people with many years of life and productivity ahead of them, and that carotid and vertebral artery dissections are responsible for approximately one-quarter of strokes in the young adult population, we propose that greater funding and efforts should be made towards research into managing the aftermath that arises from these. How can we most effectively help patients return to work? To being great parents and partners? To enjoying fulfilling qualities-of-life? When patients with these dissections have refractory pain, what is it, if anything, that alleviates their suffering the most effectively? How is anxiety in this setting alleviated? Is there any benefit to repeated imaging of the arteries over time? Should patients with dissection histories at least stay on aspirin long-term in the event of another dissection, or is the risk not justified? These are only a few of the numerous questions about long-term management after these dissections that remain unanswered.

Our intention is to update this book over time as

new studies are published. We hope that you have found the information that we have shared helpful and that something within these pages has provided better understanding for you. We thank you for reaching out by reading it!

Acknowledgements

We would like to thank the patients who have so bravely shared their stories in this book. They wished to raise carotid and vertebral artery dissection awareness by doing so, but also to provide knowledge and comfort to those who find themselves struggling through this journey. A dissection with or without stroke is a personal event that can result in a great deal of vulnerability, and we recognize that sharing the details of such a tale can feel unsettling. To those who have stepped outside of their comfort zones and put their experiences in print, we thank you.

Dianna Petty Williams spent hours editing and reading our manuscript, and we are so grateful for the polished final product she has helped us create. Dr. Edward J. Fox kindly read our manuscript and offered us some extremely helpful grammatical and editing feedback. We feel fortunate to benefit from Dr. Fox's wealth of knowledge and expertise. Linda Lauria was our first reader, and provided continuous feedback. Shreynesh Shah, MD read our manuscript so that an additional vascular neurologist could provide input. We sincerely thank everyone who sacrificed their time and shared their talents to make this book a reality.

- *Amanda P. Anderson and Jodi A. Dodds*

Acknowledgements

My interest in and appreciation for patients with carotid and vertebral artery dissections began during my neurology residency at the University of Washington, where Kyra Becker, MD, Will Longstreth, MD, David Tirschwell, MD, Sandeep Khot, MD, and Jonathan Weinstein, MD, PhD taught me a great deal about vascular injuries, patient clinical presentations, and how to manage them. I will be forever grateful to have had this experience with them at Harborview Medical Center in the acute hospital setting, as well as in the outpatient stroke specialty clinic, where my passion for caring for young stroke patients was fueled.

Richard O'Brien, MD, PhD, Chair of the Department of Neurology at Duke University, encouraged me to continue writing *The Stroke Blog* when I started at Duke in 2015. His support of my writing is so appreciated.

I cannot make enough positive comments to accurately reflect the fulfillment I get by coming to work each day at Duke, and a large part of this stems from my colleagues. Carmelo Graffagnino, MD and I have had dozens of hallway conversations about carotid and vertebral artery dissection management, and they are always thought-provoking. Kristina Balderson has answered my hundreds of research questions patiently and knowledgeably. Christa Swisher, MD and Mary Guhwe, DNP have been a continuous source of support professionally and are inspiring individuals. There are too many people to acknowledge individually, but I am grateful for the wonderful members of the Department of Neurology, the neurovascular ultrasound lab, the inpatient stroke service, and the outpatient stroke clinic who make patient care possible.

I would like to thank my brother, Tim Anderson, for his ready humor on tougher days throughout the writing process. My father and stepmother, Joe and Amanda Anderson (a different Amanda Anderson than my coauthor), have been a consistent source of encouragement and support throughout this process.

I will never be able to convey the depths of my gratitude for my mother, Helen Anderson, who has always believed in me and my dreams, and this shows through her actions. Without her love and assistance this book would not exist.

I thank my coauthor and good friend, Amanda Anderson. There were so many times along the way when I would fall away from writing as life got busy, and she always brought me back to task in a kind way. This book would not exist without her passion for the plight of patients with carotid and vertebral artery dissections, as well as her persistence. Thank you, Amanda, for getting me to the finish line.

Most importantly, I sincerely thank the patients with carotid and vertebral artery dissections who have entrusted me with their care. You are an inspiring group of people, and it means the world to me that you have chosen me as your partner in guiding you through your aftermath. I have learned a great deal from you.

- *Jodi A. Dodds, MD*

[1] Image Source:Anatomy & Physiology, Arteries Supplying the Head and Neck" by Phil Schatz. License CC-BY https://www.lecturio.com/magazine/neuroanatomy-blood-supply-brain/

[2] The American Heart Association (2014) Types of Strokes. Retrieved from http://www.strokeassociation.org/STROKEORG/AboutStroke/TypesofStroke/Types-of-Stroke_UCM_308531_SubHomePage.jsp

[3] Stroke. (2017, May 09). Retrieved July 02, 2017, from https://www.cdc.gov/stroke/facts.htm

[4] IImage Source:Anatomy & Physiology, "Cirle of Willis"" by Phil Schatz. License CC-BY https://www.lecturio.com/magazine/neuroanatomy-blood-supply-brain/

[5] Blumenfeld, Hal, MD, PhD. Neuroanatomy through Clinical Cases. Sunderland, M.A.: Sinauer, 2002. Print.

[6] Krabbe-Hartkamp MJ, van der Grond J, de Leeuw FE, de Groot JC, Algra A, Hillen B, Breteler MM, Mali WP. "Circle of Willis: morphologic variation of three-dimensional time-of-flight MR angiograms." Radiology 1998 Apr; 207(1): 103-11.

[7] Image Source: Grey's Anatomy 1918 CC-BY via: https://commons.wikimedia.org/wiki/File:Arteries_beneath_brain.png

[8] Haneline, M., & Rosner, A. (2007, August 1). The etiology of cervical artery dissection. Retrieved January 3, 2016, from http://www.ncbi.nlm.nih.gov/pmc/articles/PMC2647091/

[9] Image Source: BruceBlaus, https://en.wikipedia.org/wiki/Tunica_media#/media/File:Blausen_0055_ArteryWallStructure.pn g CC-BY 3.0.

[10] Haneline, M. T., & Rosner, A. L. (2007). The etiology of cervical artery dissection. Journal of Chiropractic Medicine, 6(3), 110-120. doi:10.1016/j.jcme.2007.04.007

[11] Wilkinson Iain M. The Vertebral Artery: Extracranial and Intracranial Structure. Arch Neurol. 1972; 27(5):392-6.

[12] Dodds, J. The Stroke Blog. Oct 8, 2014.

[13] Image Source: CC-BY. https://www.nhibi.nih.gov/health-topics/topics/catd

[14] Image Source: College of Human Medicine, Michigan State University CC-BY,, via: https://openi.nlm.nih.gov/detailedresult.php?img=PMC3774994_fneur-04-00133-g001&query=artery+dissection&it=g&req=4&npos=31

[15] Zohrabian, MD, FAAEM, D. (2015, September 2). Carotid Artery Dissection (B. Brenner, MD, PhD, FACEP, Ed.). Retrieved January 5, 2016, from http://emedicine.medscape.com/article/757906-overview#a6

[16] Blum, C., & Yaghi, S. (2015). Cervical Artery Dissection: A Review of the Epidemiology, Pathophysiology, Treatment, and Outcome. Arch Neurosci Archives of Neuroscience.

[17] Steinsiepe VK, Jung S, Goeggel Simonetti B and Arnold M. Spontaneous Cervical Artery Dissection. Austin J Clin Neurol 2014;1(3): 1012.

[18] Blum, C., & Yaghi, S. (2015). Cervical Artery Dissection: A Review of the Epidemiology, Pathophysiology, Treatment, and Outcome. Arch Neurosci Archives of Neuroscience.

[19] Steinsiepe VK, Jung S, Goeggel Simonetti B and Arnold M. Spontaneous Cervical Artery Dissection. Austin J Clin Neurol 2014;1(3): 1012.

[20] Blum, C., & Yaghi, S. (2015). Cervical Artery Dissection: A Review of the Epidemiology, Pathophysiology, Treatment, and Outcome. Arch Neurosci Archives of Neuroscience.l.

[21] Schievink, W. I. (2001). Spontaneous Dissection of the Carotid and Vertebral Arteries. *New England Journal of Medicine, 344*(12), 898-906. doi:10.1056/nejm200103223441206

[22] Debette, S. et al. Common variation in PHACTR1 is associated with susceptibility to cervical artery dissection. Nature Genetics, 2014.

[23] Shea K, Stahmer S. Carotid and vertebral arterial dissections in the emergency department. Emerg Med Pract. 2012 Apr;14(4):1-23.

[24] Image Source: CC-BY via: https://commons.wikimedia.org/wiki/File:StrokeMCA_overlay.png

[25] Phea K, Stahmer S. Carotid and vertebral arterial dissections in the

[26] Shea K, Stahmer S. Carotid and vertebral arterial dissections in the emergency department. Emerg Med Pract. 2012 Apr;14(4):1-23.

[27] Campos-Herrera, C., Scaff, M., Yamamoto, F., & Conforto, A. (n.d.). Spontaneous cervical artery dissection: An update on clinical and diagnostic aspects. Arq. Neuro-Psiquiatr. Arquivos De Neuro-Psiquiatria,922-927.

[28] Source:Gray's Anatomy, Via https://commons.wikimedia.org/wiki/File:Anatomy,_descriptive_and_surgical_(1897)_(14 5783 01709).jpg, CC-BY.

[29] Blum, C., & Yaghi, S. (2015). Cervical Artery Dissection: A Review of the Epidemiology, Pathophysiology, Treatment, and Outcome. Arch Neurosci Archives of Neuroscience.

[30] Peterson, Aldeen, & Solomon. (2013). Focus On: Headache and Neck Pain–When to Suspect Cervical ... Retrieved February 02, 2016, from http://www.acep.org/Education/Continuing-Medical-Education-(CME)/Focus-On/Focus-On--H eadache-and-Neck-Pain---When-to-Suspect-Cervical-Artery-Dissection/.

[31] Image Source, CC-BY via: https://commons.wikimedia.org/wiki/File:Cervical_XRayFlexionExtension.jpg

[32] Steinsiepe VK, Jung S, Goeggel Simonetti B and Arnold M. Spontaneous Cervical Artery Dissection. Austin J Clin Neurol 2014;1(3): 1012.

[33] Peterson, Aldeen, & Solomon. (2013). Focus On: Headache and Neck Pain–When to Suspect Cervical ... Retrieved February 02, 2016, from http://www.acep.org/Education/Continuing-Medical-Education-(CME)/Focus-On/Focus-On--H eadache-and-Neck-Pain---When-to-Suspect-Cervical-Artery-Dissection/.

[34] Shea K, Stahmer S. Carotid and vertebral arterial dissections in the emergency department. Emerg Med Pract. 2012 Apr;14(4):1-23.

[35] Dodds, Jodi. "What does 'blurry vision' really mean after stroke?" *The Stroke Blog*. 29 Jan 2016. http://strokeblog.net

[36] Arnold, M., & Bousser, M. (2005). Carotid and vertebral artery dissection. *Practical Neurology, 5*(2), 100-109. doi:10.1111/j.1474-7766.2005.00292.x

[37] Peterson, Aldeen, & Solomon. (2013). Focus On: Headache and Neck Pain–When to Suspect Cervical ... Retrieved February 02, 2016, from http://www.acep.org/Education/Continuing-Medical-Education-(CME)/Focus-On/Focus-On--H eadache-and-Neck-Pain---When-to-Suspect-Cervical-Artery-Dissection/.

[38] Lyrer, P. A., Brandt, T., Metso, T. M., Metso, A. J., Kloss, M., Debette, S., . . . Grond-Ginsbach, C. (2014). Clinical import of Horner syndrome in internal carotid and vertebral artery dissection. *Neurology, 82*(18), 1653-1659. doi:10.1212/wnl.0000000000000381

[39] Borgman, C. (n.d.). Horner syndrome secondary to internal carotid artery dissection after a short-distance endurance run: A case study and review. Journal of Optometry, 209-216.

[40] Image Source: CC-BY via: https://openi.nlm.nih.gov/detailedresult.php?img=PMC545208_pmed.0020019.g001&query=horner+syndrome&it=xg&req=4&npos=2

[41] image Source: Bluemoon 538, CC-BY, via:https://commons.wikimedia.org/wiki/File:Example_of_Horner%27s_syndrome_in_a_cat.jp g

[42] Shigematsu, K., Shimamura, O., Nakano, H., Watanabe, Y., Sekimoto, T., Shimizu, K., . . . Makino, M. (2012). Vomiting should be a prompt predictor of stroke outcome. Emergency Medicine Journal, 728-731.

[43] Biller, J., Sacco, R., Albuquerque, F., Demaerschalk, B., Fayad, P., Long, P., . . . Tirschwell, D. (2014). Cervical Arterial Dissections and Association With Cervical Manipulative Therapy: A Statement for Healthcare Professionals From the American Heart Association/American Stroke Association. *Stroke,* 3155-3174.

[44] Peterson, Aldeen, & Solomon. (2013). Focus On: Headache and Neck Pain–When to Suspect Cervical ... Retrieved February 02, 2016, from http://www.acep.org/Education/Continuing-Medical-Education-(CME)/Focus-On/Focus-On--Headache-and-Neck-Pain---When-to-Suspect-Cervical-Artery-Dissection/.

[45] Vertinsky, A., Schwartz, N., Fischbein, N., Rosenberg, J., Albers, G., & Zaharchuk, G. (2008). Comparison of Multidetector CT Angiography and MR Imaging of Cervical Artery Dissection. *American Journal of Neuroradiology,* 1753-1760.

[46] Vertinsky, A., Schwartz, N., Fischbein, N., Rosenberg, J., Albers, G., & Zaharchuk, G. (2008). Comparison of Multidetector CT Angiography and MR Imaging of Cervical Artery Dissection. *American Journal of Neuroradiology,* 1753-1760.

[47] Biller, J., Sacco, R., Albuquerque, F., Demaerschalk, B., Fayad, P., Long, P., . . . Tirschwell, D. (2014). Cervical Arterial Dissections and Association With Cervical Manipulative Therapy: A Statement for Healthcare Professionals From the American Heart Association/American Stroke Association. *Stroke,* 3155-3174.

[48] Peterson, Aldeen, & Solomon. (2013). Focus On: Headache and Neck Pain–When to Suspect Cervical ... Retrieved February 02, 2016, from http://www.acep.org/Education/Continuing-Medical-Education-(CME)/Focus-On/Focus-On--Headache-and-Neck-Pain---When-to-Suspect-Cervical-Artery-Dissection/.

[49] Naggara, O., Louillet, F., Touze, E., Roy, D., Leclerc, X., Mas, J. L., . . . Oppenheim, C. (2010). Added Value of High-Resolution MR Imaging in the Diagnosis of Vertebral Artery Dissection. *American Journal of Neuroradiology, 31*(9), 1707-1712. doi:10.3174/ajnr.a2165

[50] Naggara, O., Louillet, F., Touze, E., Roy, D., Leclerc, X., Mas, J. L., . . . Oppenheim, C. (2010). Added Value of High-Resolution MR Imaging in the Diagnosis of Vertebral Artery Dissection. *American Journal of Neuroradiology, 31*(9), 1707-1712. doi:10.3174/ajnr.a216

[51] Leffers AM, Wagner A. Neurologic complications of cerebral angiography. A retrospective study of complication rate and patient risk factors. *ACT-A Radiol.* 2000 May; 41(3): 204-10.

[52] Peterson, Aldeen, & Solomon. (2013). Focus On: Headache and Neck Pain–When to Suspect Cervical ... Retrieved February 02, 2016, from

http://www.acep.org/Education/Continuing-Medical-Education-(CME)/Focus-On/Focus-On--Headache-and-Neck-Pain---When-to-Suspect-Cervical-Artery-Dissection/.
[53] Image Source: Miller, S. CC-BY.
via:https://openi.nlm.nih.gov/detailedresult.php?img=2783048_1752-1947-3-107-2&query=vertebral+artery+dissection&it=xg&req=4&npos=18
[54] Biller, J., Sacco, R., Albuquerque, F., Demaerschalk, B., Fayad, P., Long, P., . . . Tirschwell, D. (2014). Cervical Arterial Dissections and Association With Cervical Manipulative Therapy: A Statement for Healthcare Professionals From the American Heart Association/American Stroke Association. *Stroke*, 3155-3174.
[55] Image Source: National Heart Lung and Blood Institute, 12 November 2013, 21:17:20

[56] Biller, J., Sacco, R., Albuquerque, F., Demaerschalk, B., Fayad, P., Long, P., . . . Tirschwell, D. (2014). Cervical Arterial Dissections and Association With Cervical Manipulative Therapy: A Statement for Healthcare Professionals From the American Heart Association/American Stroke Association. *Stroke*, 3155-3174.
[57] Dziewas, R., Konrad, C., Dr♦Ger, B., Evers, S., Besselmann, M., LUDemann, P., . . . Ringelstein, E. (2003). Cervical artery dissection?clinical features, risk factors, therapy and outcome in 126 patients.*Journal of Neurology*, 1179-1184.
[58] Fisher, C. (n.d.). The Headache and Pain of Spontaneous Carotid Dissection. *Headache Headache: The Journal of Head and Face Pain*, 60-65.
[59] Fibromuscular Dysplasia (FMD). (2014, April 1). Retrieved January 12, 2016, from http://www.strokeassociation.org/STROKEORG/StrokeConnectionMagazine/ReadSCNow/Fibromuscular-Dysplasia-FMD_UCM_461419_Article.jsp#.VpVrePkrLq4
[60] Image source: CC-BY
https://openi.nlm.nih.gov/detailedresult.php?img=493280_1476-7120-2-7-1&query=fibromuscular+dysplasia+carotid&it=xg&req=4&npos=17
[61] Fibromuscular Dysplasia (FMD): Causes, Types, Symptoms and Treatment. (n.d.). Retrieved January 12, 2016, from http://my.clevelandclinic.org/services/heart/disorders/fibromuscular_dysplasia
[62] Kubota, I. (n.d.). Endovascular Therapy for Fibromuscular Dysplasia of the Bilateral External Iliac Arteries Visualized with Optical Coherence Tomography. *Am J Case Rep American Journal of Case Reports*, 187-190.
[63] Dziewas, R., Konrad, C., Dr♦Ger, B., Evers, S., Besselmann, M., LUDemann, P., . . . Ringelstein, E. (2003). Cervical artery dissection?clinical features, risk factors, therapy and outcome in 126 patients.*Journal of Neurology*, 1179-1184.
[64] Kadian-Dodov, D., Gornik, H. L., Gu, X., Froehlich, J., Bacharach, J. M., Chi, Y., . . . Olin, J. W. (2016). Dissection and Aneurysm in Patients With Fibromuscular Dysplasia. *Journal of the American College of Cardiology, 68*(2), 176-185. doi:10.1016/j.jacc.2016.04.044
[65] McKusick, Victor and Hamosh, Ada. Online Mendelian Inheritance in Man ("OMIM"), entry #130050.
[66] Image Source: Dagger997 CC-BY, via: https://commons.wikimedia.org/wiki/File:Fingersnake.JPG
[67] What are the signs? (n.d.). Retrieved January 13, 2016, from http://www.marfan.org/about/signs
[68] Fast Facts - Osteogenesis ImperfeCT-A Foundation | OIF.org. (n.d.). Retrieved January 13, 2016, from http://www.oif.org/site/PageServer?pagename=fastfacts
[69] Pezzini, A., Zotto, E. D., Giossi, A., Volonghi, I., Costa, P., Volta, G. D., & Padovani, A. (2011). The Migraine-Ischemic Stroke Relation in Young Adults. *Stroke Research and Treatment, 2011*, 1-7.

[70] "What Women Need To Know About The Hidden Risk Factors For Stroke," Stroke Connection Magazine, November/December 2004.
[71] James, A., MD. (n.d.). Women's Health - Blood Clots. Retrieved November 04, 2016, from https://www.stoptheclot.org/learn_more/womens_health_faq.htm
[72] Biller, J., Sacco, R., Albuquerque, F., Demaerschalk, B., Fayad, P., Long, P., . . . Tirschwell, D. (2014). Cervical Arterial Dissections and Association With Cervical
[73] Dziewas, R., Konrad, C., Dr Ger, B., Evers, S., Besselmann, M., L Demann, P., . . . Ringelstein, E. (2003). Cervical artery dissection?clinical features, risk factors, therapy and outcome in 126 patients.Journal of Neurology, 1179-1184.
[74] Dziewas, R., Konrad, C., Dr Ger, B., Evers, S., Besselmann, M., L Demann, P., . . . Ringelstein, E. (2003). Cervical artery dissection?clinical features, risk factors, therapy and outcome in 126 patients.Journal of Neurology, 1179-1184.
[75] Dziewas, R., Konrad, C., Dr Ger, B., Evers, S., Besselmann, M., L Demann, P., . . . Ringelstein, E. (2003). Cervical artery dissection?clinical features, risk factors, therapy and outcome in 126 patients.Journal of Neurology, 1179-1184.
[76] Chen, W. (2006). Vertebral artery dissection and cerebellar infarction following chiropractic manipulation. Emergency Medicine Journal.
[77] Klougart, & Leboeuf-Yde C,. (1996, July/August). Safety in chiropractic practice, Part I; The occurrence of cerebrovascular accidents after manipulation to the neck in Denmark from 1978-1988. *J Manipulative Physiol Ther, 19*(6), 371-377.
[78] Berger, S. (2014, January 6). How Safe Are the Vigorous Neck Manipulations Done by Chiropractors? The Washington Post. Retrieved January 17, 2016, from http://www.highbeam.com/doc/1P2-35557778.html?
[79] Jones, J., Jones, C., & Nugent, K. (2015, January). Vertebral artery dissection after a chiropractor neck manipulation. *Baylor University Medical Center Proceedings,28*(1), 88-90.
[80] Jones, J., Jones, C., & Nugent, K. (2015, January). Vertebral artery dissection after a chiropractor neck manipulation. *Baylor University Medical Center Proceedings,28*(1), 88-90.
[81] ACA Responds to AHA Statement on Neck Manipulation. Business Wire. 7 August 2014.
[82] Carprieaux, M., Michotte, A., Varenbergh, D. V., & Marichal, M. P. (2012). Spontaneous bilateral carotid artery dissection following cervical manipulation. *Legal Medicine, 14*(5), 249-251. doi:10.1016/j.legalmed.2012.04.002
[83] Schievink, W. I. (2000). The treatment of spontaneous carotid and vertebral artery dissections. *Current Opinion in Cardiology, 15*(5), 316-321.
[84] Rubinstein, S. M., Peerdeman, S. M., Tulder, M. W., Riphagen, I., & Haldeman, S. (2005). A Systematic Review of the Risk Factors for Cervical Artery Dissection. *Stroke, 36*(7), 1575-1580.
[85] Shea K, Stahmer S. Carotid and vertebral arterial dissections in the emergency department. Emerg Med Pract. 2012 Apr;14(4):1-23.
[86] Shea K, Stahmer S. Carotid and vertebral arterial dissections in the emergency department. Emerg Med Pract. 2012 Apr;14(4):1-23.
[87] Juszkat, R., Liebert, W., Stanisławska, K., Tomczyk, T., Wronka, J., Wąsik, N., & Perek, B. (2015). Extracranial Internal Carotid Artery Dissection Treated with Self-expandable Stents: A Single-Centre Experience.*CardioVascular and Interventional Radiology Cardiovasc Intervent Radiol, 38*(6), 1451-1457.

[88] Shea K, Stahmer S. Carotid and vertebral arterial dissections in the emergency department. Emerg Med Pract. 2012 Apr;14(4):1-23.
[89] Menon, R. K., & Norris, J. W. (2008). Cervical Arterial Dissection. *Annals of the New York Academy of Sciences, 1142*(1), 200-217.
[90] Shanmugalingam, R., Pour, N. R., Chuah, S. C., Vo, T. M., Beran, R., Hennessy, A., & Makris, A. (2016). Vertebral artery dissection in hypertensive disorders of pregnancy: A case series and literature review. *BMC Pregnancy and Childbirth,16*(1). doi:10.1186/s12884-016-0953-5
[91] Stamboulis, E., Raptis, G., Andrikopoulou, A., Arvaniti, C., Brountzos, E., Oikonomopoulos, N., . . . Voumvourakis, K. (2010). Spontaneous Internal Carotid Artery Dissection: An Uncommon Cause of Recurrent PostPArtum Headache. *Journal of Neuroimaging, 21*(1), 76-78. doi:10.1111/j.1552-6569.2009.00387.x
[92] Shea K, Stahmer S. Carotid and vertebral arterial dissections in the emergency department. Emerg Med Pract. 2012 Apr;14(4):1-23.

[93] Shea K, Stahmer S. Carotid and vertebral arterial dissections in the emergency department. Emerg Med Pract. 2012 Apr;14(4):1-23.
I.
[94] Image Source: DR. Johannes Sobotta, CC-BY, via: https://commons.wikimedia.org/wiki/File:Sobo_1909_550.png
[95] Shea K, Stahmer S. Carotid and vertebral arterial dissections in the emergency department. Emerg Med Pract. 2012 Apr;14(4):1-23.
[96] Fisher, C. (n.d.). The Headache and Pain of Spontaneous Carotid Dissection. *Headache Headache: The Journal of Head and Face Pain*, 60-65.
[97] Chimowitz, M., Lynn, M., & Howlett-Smith, H. (2005). Comparison of Warfarin and Aspirin for Symptomatic Intracranial Arterial Stenosis. *ACC Current Journal Review, 14*(8), 20. doi:10.1016/j.accreview.2005.08.035
[98] Stroke Treatments. (n.d.). Retrieved January 17, 2016, from http://www.strokeassociation.org/STROKEORG/AboutStroke/Treatment/Stroke-Treatments_UCM_310892_Article.jsp#.Vpwf6fkrLq4

[99] Massop, D., Dave, R., Metzger, C., Bachinsky, W., Solis, M., Shah, R., . . . Hibbard, R. (2009). Stenting and Angioplasty with Protection in Patients at High-Risk for Endarterectomy: SAPPHIRE Worldwide Registry First 2,001 Patients. *Catheterization and Cardiovascular Interventions, 73*(2), 129-136. doi:10.1002/ccd.21844
[100] Brott,, T. G., & Et al. (2010). Stenting versus Endarterectomy for Treatment of Carotid-Artery Stenosis. *New England Journal of Medicine, 363*(2), 198-198. doi:10.1056/nejmx100035
[101] Hacke, W. (1995). Intravenous Thrombolysis With Recombinant Tissue Plasminogen Activator for Acute Hemispheric Stroke. *Jama, 274*(13), 1017. doi:10.1001/jama.1995.03530130023023
[102] Tissue Plasminogen Activator for Acute Ischemic Stroke. (1995). *New England Journal of Medicine, 333*(24), 1581-1588. doi:10.1056/nejm199512143332401
[103] Keyser, J. D., Gdovinova, Z., Uyttenboogaart, M., Vroomen, P. C., & Luijckx, G. J. (2007). Intravenous Alteplase for Stroke: Beyond the Guidelines and in Particular Clinical Situations. *Stroke, 38*(9), 2612-2618.
[104] Steinsiepe VK, Jung S, Goeggel Simonetti B and Arnold M. Spontaneous Cervical Artery Dissection. Austin J Clin Neurol 2014;1(3): 1012.

[105] Steinsiepe VK, Jung S, Goeggel Simonetti B and Arnold M. Spontaneous Cervical Artery Dissection. Austin J Clin Neurol 2014;1(3): 1012.
[106] Steinsiepe VK, Jung S, Goeggel Simonetti B and Arnold M. Spontaneous Cervical Artery Dissection. Austin J Clin Neurol 2014;1(3): 1012.
[107] Mustanoja, S., Metso, T., Putaala, J., Heikkinen, N., Haapaniemi, E., Salonen, O., & Tatlisumak, T. (2015). Helsinki experience on nonvitamin K oral anticoagulants for treating cervical artery dissection. *Brain Behav Brain and Behavior.*
[108] *The Scream* [Photograph of painting]. (1893). The National Gallery, Oslo In E. Munch (Author).
[109] Baumgartner R.W., Arnold M., Baumgartner I. Carotid dissection with and without ischemic events: local symptoms and cerebral artery findings. Neurology. 2001;57(5):827–832.
[110] Lithograph, 1853, CC-BY.
[111] Image Source: Kang, CC-BY, https://openi.nlm.nih.gov/detailedresult.php?img=PMC4040639_kjs-10-249-g003&query=carotid+artery+cranial+nerves&it=xg&req=4&npos=4
[112] Fisher, C. M. (1982). The Headache and Pain of Spontaneous Carotid Dissection.*Headache Headache: The Journal of Head and Face Pain, 22*(2), 60-65.
[113] Trigeminal Neuralgia Fact Shee. (n.d.). Retrieved December 05, 2016, from http://www.ninds.nih.gov/disorders/trigeminal_neuralgia/detail_trigeminal_neuralgia.html
[114] The American Association of Neurological Surgeons. (n.d.). Retrieved December 05, 2016, from http://www.aans.org/patient information/conditions and treatments/trigeminal neuralgia.aspx
[115] "Teaching the Nervous System to Forget Chronic Pain." *PBS.* Public Broadcasting Service, 13 Feb. 2015. Web. 28 May 2017.
[116] Biller, J., Sacco, R., Albuquerque, F., Demaerschalk, B., Fayad, P., Long, P., . . . Tirschwell, D. (2014). Cervical Arterial Dissections and Association With Cervical Manipulative Therapy: A Statement for Healthcare Professionals From the American Heart Association/American Stroke Association. *Stroke,* 3155-3174.

[117] Strauss, L. D., Weizenbaum, E., Loder, E. W., & Rizzoli, P. B. (2016). Amitriptyline Dose and Treatment Outcomes in Specialty Headache Practice: A Retrospective Cohort Study. *Headache: The Journal of Head and Face Pain, 56*(10), 1626-1634. doi:10.1111/head.12987
[118] Peggy Peck Peggy Peck. (2006). FDA Warns on Mixing Antidepressants with Migraine Drugs. Retrieved December 29, 2016, from http://www.medpagetoday.com/Neurology/Migraines/3770
[119] Blumenfeld A., Ashkenazi A., Grosberg B., Napehan U., Narouze S., Nett B., Lipton R. (2010). Patterns of use of peripheral nerve blocks and trigger point injections among headache practitioners in the USA: Results of the American headache society interventional procedure survey (AHS-IPS). Headache, 50, 937–942. doi:10.1111/j.1526–4610.2010.01676.x

[120] Image Source CC_BY via: https://openi.nlm.nih.gov/detailedresult.php?img=PMC4235127_SNI-5-155-g001&query=occipital+nerve+&req=4&npos=63
[121] Greater Occipital Nerve Block Hopkins Medicine. (n.d.). Retrieved February 2, 16, from

http://www.hopkinsmedicine.org/neurology_neurosurgery/centers_clinics/headache/procedures/greater_occipital_nerve_block.html

[122] Millstine, D., Chen, C. Y., & Bauer, B. (2017). Complementary and integrative medicine in the management of headache. *Bmj*. doi:10.1136/bmj.j1805

[123] Linde, K., Allais, G., Brinkhaus, B., Manheimer, E., Vickers, A., & White, A. R. (2015). Acupuncture for migraine prophylaxis. *Sao Paulo Medical Journal, 133*(6), 540-540. doi:10.1590/1516-3180.20151336t1

[124] Chen, Y., & Wang, H. (2014). The Effectiveness of Acupressure on Relieving Pain: A Systematic Review. *Pain Management Nursing, 15*(2), 539-550. doi:10.1016/j.pmn.2012.12.005

[125] Hsieh, L. L., Liou, H., Lee, L., Chen, T. H., & Yen, A. M. (2010). Effect of Acupressure and Trigger Points in Treating Headache: A Randomized Controlled Trial. *The American Journal of Chinese Medicine Am. J. Chin. Med., 38*(01), 1-14. doi:10.1142/s0192415x10007634

[126] 49. doi:10.1016/j.mehy.2009.11.037Blunt, S. B., & Lee, H. P. (2010). Can traditional "cupping" treatment cause a stroke? *Medical Hypotheses, 74*(5), 945-9

[127] Choi, J. Y., Huh, C. W., Choi, C. H., & Lee, J. I. (2016). Extracranial vertebral artery rupture likely secondary to "cupping therapy" superimposed on spontaneous dissection. *Interventional Neuroradiology*. doi:10.1177/1591019916659264

[128] Ament Headache Center | Botox for Migraines, Migraine Relief. (n.d.). Retrieved January 26, 2016, from http://www.amentheadachecenter.com/headaches/botox/

[129] Lee, M., Silverman, S., Hansen, H., Patel, V., & Manchikanti, L. (2011). A comprehensive review of opioid-induced hyperalgesia. *Pain Physician, 14*(2), 145-161

[130] UNODC, World Drug Report 2012. http://www.unodc.org/unodc/en/data-and-analysis/WDR-2012.html

[131] Sasannejad, P., Saeedi, M., Shoeibi, A., Gorji, A., Abbasi, M., & Foroughipour, M. (2012). Lavender Essential Oil in the Treatment of Migraine Headache: A Placebo-Controlled Clinical Trial. *European Neurology Eur Neurol, 67*(5), 288-291.

[132] Maghbooli, M., Golipour, F., Esfandabadi, A. M., & Yousefi, M. (2013). Comparison Between the Efficacy of Ginger and Sumatriptan in the Ablative Treatment of the Common Migraine. *Phytotherapy Research, 28*(3), 412-415. doi:10.1002/ptr.4996

[133] Sampson, S. R., & Weiss-Rotem, C. (1982). RELAXANT EFFECTS OF LITHIUM ON GUINEA-PIG TRACHEAL SMOOTH MUSCLE in vitro. *British Journal of Pharmacology, 75*(2), 287-291.

[134] Image source: CC-BY, via: https://commons.wikimedia.org/wiki/File:Gray779.png

[135] Edmondson, D., Richardson, S., Fausett, J. K., Falzon, L., Howard, V. J., & Kronish, I. M. (2013). Prevalence of PTSD in Survivors of Stroke and Transient Ischemic Attack: A Meta-Analytic Review. *PLoS ONE, 8*(6). doi:10.1371/journal.pone.0066435

[136] Post-Traumatic Stress Disorder after Stroke – Flint Rehab. Retrieved November 08, 2016, from https://www.flintrehab.com/2016/post-traumatic-stress-disorder-after-stroke/

[137] Edmondson, D., Richardson, S., Fausett, J. K., Falzon, L., Howard, V. J., & Kronish, I. M. (2013). Prevalence of PTSD in Survivors of Stroke and Transient Ischemic Attack: A Meta-Analytic Review. *PLoS ONE, 8*(6). doi:10.1371/journal.pone.0066435

[138] Kronish, I. M., Edmondson, D., Goldfinger, J. Z., Fei, K., & Horowitz, C. R. (2012). Posttraumatic Stress Disorder and Adherence to Medications in Survivors of Strokes and Transient Ischemic Attacks. *Stroke, 43*(8), 2192-2197. doi:10.1161/strokeaha.112.655209

[139] A Mini-Stroke Called A TIA Can Spark Post-Traumatic Stress. (n.d.). Retrieved November 11, 2016, from http://www.npr.org/sections/health-shots/2014/10/02/353202992/a-mini-stroke-called-a-tia-can-spark-post-traumatic-stress

[140] Speck, V., Noble, A., Kollmar, R., & Schenk, T. (2014). Diagnosis of Spontaneous Cervical Artery Dissection May Be Associated with Increased Prevalence of Posttraumatic Stress Disorder. *Journal of Stroke and Cerebrovascular Diseases,23*(2), 335-342. doi:10.1016/j.jstrokecerebrovasdis.2013.03.033

[141] Fatigue. (2014). Retrieved November 11, 2016, from http://www.stroke.org/we-can-help/survivors/stroke-recovery/post-stroke-conditions/physical/fatigue

[142] Hoffer, M. E., Szczupak, M., Kiderman, A., Crawford, J., Murphy, S., Marshall, K., . . . Balaban, C. (2016). Neurosensory Symptom Complexes after Acute Mild Traumatic Brain Injury. *PLOS ONE PLoS ONE, 11*(1).

[143] Maaijwee, N. A., Arntz, R. M., Rutten-Jacobs, L. C., Schaapsmeerders, P., Schoonderwaldt, H. C., Dijk, E. J., & Leeuw, F. D. (2014). Post-stroke fatigue and its association with poor functional outcome after stroke in young adults.*Journal of Neurology, Neurosurgery & Psychiatry J Neurol Neurosurg Psychiatry,86*(10), 1120-1126. doi:10.1136/jnnp-2014-308784

[144] Smith, E. E., Schneider, J. A., Wardlaw, J. M., & Greenberg, S. M. (2012). Cerebral microinfarcts: the invisible lesions. *The Lancet Neurology, 11*(3), 272-282. doi:10.1016/s1474-4422(11)70307-6

[145] Social Security. (n.d.). Retrieved December 30, 2016, from https://www.ssa.gov/planners/disability/dqualify4.html

[146] Kim, S., Lee, Y., Suh, S., Lee, J., Ryu, K., & Kang, D. (2016). Acute Pontine Infarction due to Basilar Artery Dissection from Strenuous Physical Effort: One from Sexual Intercourse and Another from Defecation. *Journal of Cerebrovascular and Endovascular Neurosurgery, 18*(2), 100. doi:10.7461/jcen.2016.18.2.100